WORSHIP YOUR FOOD

Quinn Montana

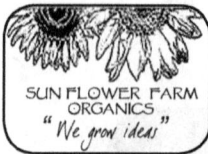

SUN FLOWER FARM
ORGANICS
" We grow ideas "

Sunflower Farm Press
POB 934
Huntsville, AR 72740
479-677-2002
onegreengrrl@hotmail.com

www.worshipyourfood.com

In Memory of

Michael J. Haden

Whose generous love and support

Allowed me the time to write this book

Acknowledgments

The following people did not necessarily help me directly in the writing of this book, all opinions and mistakes (notably the admittedly haphazard punctuation) are my own. But I wish to thank these folks for the richness they have brought to my life, because when else is one able to publicly do that? I want the world to know that you are my angels.

With eternal love and gratitude

To my sister Diane

Not only for her editing assistance and comments,
but especially for being a source of encouragement,
solace and strength throughout my life.
You are a blessing beyond measure.

And with grateful acknowledgement to all the following people whose gift of friendship has kept me alive currently and in the difficult decades preceding this writing:

Bill Fuller (my fabulous computer guru and brother-in-law) Dr. Justine Cassell, Dr. Shirley A. Gilmore, Robin Thompson, Rachel Haney, Paige Tower, Judith Keller-Hargrave, Harry and Jill Sakalares, the members of the 1990's First Existentialist Congregation of Atlanta, GA, Eileen Moremen, Holly Deal, Jean and Roy Lamer, Ann Lam, Bess Miller, Karin and Steve Stern, Jane Mahone, Karla Crawford, Gail and Bill Fuller Sr., Mary Krienke and Sarah Fuller, Lisa McCormack and Ron Giles, Barbara and David Benoit, Marty and Larry Karigan-Winter, Mike Haley and Susy Siegele, Ricky and Ginny Broyles, and the members of the Unitarian Universalist Congregation of Fayetteville, Arkansas.

Table of Contents

INTRODUCTION

Food is God

(Hindu saying)

Food is the very essence of our lives. Without sustenance we die. Without food we are nothing. We are inescapably indivisible from the plants and animals around us which we raise and eat, and which, once ingested, become us.

We have played carelessly and cavalierly with our food supply and the systems that support it for far too long. The arrogance and hubris that we have exhibited towards the fundamental wellspring of our existence is breathtaking. Food is sacred.

This disregard for our gifts, our real wealth —our soil, our seeds, the water, the air— must be considered blasphemy in any religious persuasion and morally unconscionable and ethically reprehensible to any human being regardless of belief system.

We must worship our food, and learn to approach eating with a sense of veneration, of wonder. With joy and thankfulness. We must re-learn reverence and gratitude for the meal before us; for the amazing product of rain and earthworm, sunshine and good fortune that it is.

We must, each one of us, develop the sincere desire to show homage to the living plants and animals which will make up our next meal. That something as tiny and hard as a seed could become a tree which produces an apple, all tart-sweetness, crisp, juicy and life-giving, is truly a miracle.

Today we are in the throes of a rash of epidemics in Western culture.

A precursor to many diseases is our obesity epidemic which sickens millions leaving them weak, debilitated and vulnerable to other health issues.

What is the cause of this epidemic?

> "One single apple tree can live for more than forty years and provide more than 10,000 pounds of food."
>
> (http://treesforlife.org)

The cause is simple and yet profound: We have forgotten to be grateful for our food. We have lost the spiritual bond, the thread of connection which human beings in the past have always understood intertwined our lives with the land, and with the bounty of the land.

We have lost a sense of the miraculous joy that is food.

Our bodies are a facet of the ecosystem in which we live, intricate and complex. It isn't necessary that we fully understand this complexity but that we respect it. It is imperative for us as a species and for all other species that we treat ourselves with reverence. Not the self-flattering shallow arrogance of "I deserve the best, the most expensive, most rare, most indulgent *whatever*," that has become the hallmark of Western society. The kind of reverence that, in sitting and reading, in walking, running, in being, inhales deeply and says, "I live." "I am life."

This book does not suggest a particular deity to whom one should be grateful. Only that the simple act of contemplating our food, of considering the various components in our meal and the journey through which they arrived on our plates, of spending a moment or two in recognition — in awe— of the gift of life that our food is offering to us, will be what actually saves our lives.

'The man who robs a fellow subject
of a few shillings on the highway is
sentenced to death,

but he who distributes a slow poison
to the whole community escapes
unpunished'.

Frederick Accum, 1820

CHAPTER 1

What's In *Your* Fridge?

And it came about as they were eating of the stew,
that they cried out and said,
"O man of God, there is death in the pot."

And they were unable to eat.
2 Kings 4:38-41 (Old Testament)

We live in a world of haste and waste. We rush, we run, we wolf down doughnuts while driving to work, slip in a sandwich while sitting at our desks. Our food is ubiquitous and unappreciated. It has been cheapened (literally), devalued, and is taken for granted. The amount of food discarded daily in the US would feed the entire populations of more than a third of the countries in the world.[1] And yet, Americans actually spend a smaller share of their disposable income on food than the citizens of any other country.[2] According to the U.S. Department of Agriculture, the amount Americans spend on food as a percentage of disposable income has fallen from 15.4 percent in 1980 to 10.8 percent in 2004.[3]

Entire avenues in every major city in the country are devoted to the garish vending of "cheap and quick" as a means of hastily attending to the demands of our bodies before moving on to the more important issues of either acquisition or leisure. Our food is served while we are in conversation and we typically dive in without a thought.

Rarely, if ever, does the average eater pause to consider how the food was raised; the farming methods, the fertilizers, the pesticides, the pollutants the animal or plant encountered or absorbed in it's life, the conditions under which it lived, the actual quality of the ingredients. You can't taste those things... or can you? "I've been eating that stuff for years," I've heard people say, "and I'm not dead yet." But, take a closer look— does that mean it hasn't affected you?

In an amusing episode of the television show *King of the Hill*, the family sits down to their first organic meal. They are making murmuring sounds of stunned surprise and appreciation when Peggy

Hill looks up from her plate and asks "If this is food, what have we been eating all this time?" Good question.

Quick, what did you have for dinner last night? Do you even remember? It's a question you might hear from many books that deal with one's diet. Consider this instead: Did you eat food?

It's a question so seemingly apparent that it appears laughable. Food is what we eat, right? Food is what sustains us. Food is what nourishes us. Food is life.

So how much thought have you given to the composition of the food that you eat? If a substance has no nutritional value, can it be called food? One of the chief problems we have in our modern culture is that we call anything "food" if it is edible. So, is food anything that can be eaten without killing us on the spot? According to our current standards, the answer is pretty much "yes."

A human toddler will put just about anything in its mouth. Its parents must teach it to understand that some things are edible and some are not. How do we make that distinction? After the removal of obvious poisons and dangerous substances from the list, how do we determine which things are food? It seems like a silly question, yet it has become surprisingly difficult to answer.

"Food," a mother teaching her child might say, "is what's good for us." Hmmm. Our behavior seems to contradict that.

Obviously not everything edible is nutritive or beneficial. Wood chips would fit in our mouths, but we don't eat them, per se, because we get nothing out of them. Cardboard and shoe leather and even Styrofoam can be chewed and can be swallowed in moderation without particularly ill effects, at least in the immediate. But I'll bet you would demur if offered them on a plate. Yet we ironically label nearly all things that we ingest "food," even if our diet today often contains some of those very elements.

So what else defines that which we know to be food? It seemed like such a simple thing. Of course we know it when we see it. Right?

Its something that smells good, tastes good. Something appealing, comforting, filling.

Today, that could be anything.

We even self-mockingly have a category of ingestible goods we've designated "junk food" in which we readily indulge. Many of us actually seek out laboratory concocted fake fats and fake sugars because we've been told that by eating them we might "fool" our bodies. This placing of all ingestible things under the grand moniker of "food" evolved from the not-so-distant past when an individual's meals throughout the day were made at home from actual, nutritious components. That is no longer the case. It made sense then. Today we're living in a different world.

Why is lemon juice made with artificial flavor, and dishwashing liquid made with real lemons?

It is time we stop and recognize the great chasm in our grocery stores dividing those things we evolved to eat from those which have emerged out of commercial laboratories. Laboratories whose goal it is to trick us into spending our money on cheap rip-off copies of real food, aimed at placating our taste buds (and our inner child) at huge cost to our bodies. It's as if the supermarket were a lake which contained decoy ducks floating there in the rushes amongst the few real ducks— and we are eating the decoys!

The irony is that, in choosing to remove ourselves from dung, from farm animals and soil for reasons of distain, of not getting our hands dirty, we have instead surrounded ourselves with organophosphates, carbamates, phthalates, benzene derivatives, and more. Throughout the last century, in our effort to flee the gritty labor of the farm, we have impetuously saturated our soil, our farm workers and our food with substances far worse than cow patties.

These concocted new components of mainstream food are neither nutritious nor safe. Some of them are residues of the miasma in which the product was grown or raised, as we will see, but many of the ingredients of a product, or often entire products are man-made. They are created in a lab by people whose focus is the bottom line, the next promotion, the success of a company, the enthusiasm of their stockbrokers, or sometimes simply the thrill of creating a new scientific concoction or process. The larger picture of long term health for themselves or future generations is lost to those living in the immediacy of today's Western culture.

Maybe you have already begun trying to eat well and your choices in the grocery lean more towards vegetables, meats, and meal components that you prepare yourself at home. You might be feeling that you are exempt from the issues suffered by those who subsist on fast food or junk food. If your food is conventional supermarket fare, you'd be wrong.

Archeologists have long been aware that the ancient Romans suffered conspicuously from the lead that was in their drinking and storage vessels, their plumbing, their food preservation. It has been suggested as having played a significant role in the decay and dissolution of Rome. Likewise, we're shocked and appalled when we read stories of medical patients in previous centuries being dosed with turpentine or arsenic or mercury. Well, what will future generations think when they look back on what we eat, and what it's doing to us? Even more shameful is that we knew what it was doing to us but profit seemed to be our only concern.

These are the scientifically accepted, governmentally sanctioned practices we have used, and in some cases are still using, to feed our cattle, cattle which we then used as food: Road kill, plastic bits, the waste products of other livestock, the pelletized remains of their own species, arsenic (until recent outrage stopped the practice), all have been considered legitimate feedstock by the USDA (United States Department of Agriculture.) The decision to use these non-edible, deleterious or revolting items to create food for ourselves is a decision made, not by a single lunatic king or ruler, but by dozens, hundreds, thousands of seemingly sane individuals throughout our current food production network.

4

What's In *Your* Fridge?

When you think of a cow, or a hog or a chicken, think of the skin as a wrapper containing all those ingredients and more. When you look at a steak or a chicken breast, bacon or ground meat, realize that it is a mixture of all the things that make it up, even if you can't see the individual elements. It is not grass and sunshine converted by the cow's cells into radiant, life-giving muscle meat as it was in the past. It's not acorns and roots as was the case for the hog, nor insects and seeds and chickweed and the like, as sustained chickens since the beginning of time. It's antibiotics, manure, and indigestible grains –foreign to a cow's ecological niche and foreign to its ability to break down and make use of it. And, while hogs and chickens have a broader digestive range, it's worse than mere grain or antibiotics.

Just take a look at what's being fed to the animals you eat:

Same Species Meat

Diseased Animals !

Feathers, Hair, Hooves

Urea (the main component of urine, though here it's often synthetic urea)

Manure and Other Animal Waste

Cement Dust[4]

Plastics !

Drugs and Chemicals, including formaldehyde[5], antibiotics

Genetically modified, pesticide saturated soybeans

Unhealthy Amounts of Grains* [6] (mostly GM corn, also laden with pesticides)

> *Cattle are grass eaters, they did not evolve to eat grains—the cattle are experiencing constant chronic indigestion.

As if this wasn't bad enough, until recently it was also considered "ok" to feed them roadkill collected by the county, and the diseased or euthanized bodies of dogs and cats contributed to the rendering plants by the local vets. Public outcry over fears of mad cow disease succeeded in changing those practices.

Consider also that all of our livestock animals are now eating the same diet with minor adjustments (corn, corn and corn.[7]) So, rather than various elements of our environment being taken up and utilized by diverse animals, —offering us various combinations of minerals and nutrients which may very well offer us some subtle health benefits, the way different vegetables contribute to our diets— now, beneath the skin of every livestock animal exists nearly the same concocted swampmud wreaking havoc on their bodies on the way to wreaking havoc on ours. And thus we have noxious diseased rotting (but walking!) animals which are entering our food supply— requiring ever larger government meat recalls, after you've eaten the meat.

Of course, not all items in your local grocery store come from animals. Here are some of the many products that come from... wood:

sandwich bags	stain remover	filters
coffee filters	cologne	rayon clothing
tissues	solvents	adhesives
disposable diapers	**baby food**	floor tiles
hair spray	**imitation bacon**	toothpaste
building insulation	**cereals**	helmets/hardhats
furniture	explosives	luggage
charcoal	**vegetarian foods**	plastic twines
cork	**baked goods**	cleaning agents
shoe polish	**beverages**	ceramics
cosmetics	sanding sealers	deodorant
oil spill control agents	**food additives**	fungicides
garden mulch	**food thickeners**	insecticides
grouting	**vanilla flavoring**	crayons

Source: South Carolina Forestry Association
http://www.scforestry.org/wood/treasure.html

Look at the list above. These products are being synthesized out of wood pulp: Imitation bacon, baked goods, cereals. Baby food! According to the American Gastroenterological Association (AGA), Americans report more than 81 million cases of chronic digestive problems each year.[8] The incidence of reflux in children between the ages of 2 and 17 years of age was found to have risen by 30-50% just between 2000 and 2005. Infants have experienced a 262% rise in the incidence (the number of new occurrences in the population) of reflux over the same time period.[9]

Do we wonder why? I have a solution: stop eating the wooden decoys and eat real food!

Vegetarians are not exempt from these toxic treats. As seen above, some vegetarian products are also constructed out of wood pulp, among other laboratory amalgamations. Here's another tasty example:

> According to the US EPA, Adipic acid (C6H10O4) is a white crystalline solid used *primarily as the main constituent of nylon* (nylon-6/6), representing about half of the nylon molecule. It is also used in the manufacture of some low-temperature synthetic lubricants, synthetic fibers, coatings, plastics, polyurethane resins, and plasticizers, **and to give some imitation food products a tangy flavor** and as an acidity regulator.[10] (my emphasis)

Soy protein isolate, nowadays a ubiquitous component of not only vegetarian diets but found in up to 60% of processed foods according to researchers at Cornell University [11], was originally introduced to American industry as a binder and sealer for cardboard boxes.

It is now part of nearly every processed food that you'll find on your shelves. It is in many supplements and vitamins (vitamin E can be derived from soy oil), and in foods as diverse as canned tuna, chocolate, sauces, baked goods, meat (injected under poultry skin), soups and in skin care products and pet food.[12]

> "It was approved for packaging but it was never given GRAS [generally regarded as safe] status. It hasn't actually been approved as a food ingredient." says Kaayla Daniel, PhD, clinical nutritionist and author of *The Whole Soy Story: The Dark Side of America's Favorite Health Food.*

In addition, ninety percent of all soy grown has been genetically modified. What does that mean? According to the previous Cornell University source:

"All plants and animals have DNA, and use their DNA-based instructions called genes to make proteins. A genetically engineered plant carries one or more new genes, and usually (but not always) makes a new protein. These two additions— the new gene(s) and the new protein(s)— are the 'new' parts **that consumers are eating**. (my emphasis)

Genes are the instructions all living things use to build and maintain their cells. Adding a new gene to a crop may give it a trait that is useful to growers and consumers, making plants that are more resistant to insects and disease, that simplify weed control, or that produce fruits with longer shelf life."

In the case of the soybean, the genetic modification allows the plant to be saturated with a lethal amount of the herbicide RoundUp, to absorb that toxic cocktail into its cells and still remain alive.[13] This means that those plants are imbued throughout their cells with Monsanto's chemicals—they won't wash off. The FDA (Food and Drug Administration) is trying to convince you that this is a good thing. Meanwhile, according to USDA data, the soybean is the domestic crop most contaminated with controversial organophosphate pesticides.[14]

Plants, like humans, store toxins in lipid (fat) cells, so of all the foods containing toxins that we ingest, the worst possible ones are the ones containing the most fats/ oils. Soybean oil accounts for 79 percent of the edible fats used annually in the United States, according to the United Soybean Board.[15] And we've just seen that soybeans are the domestic crop most contaminated with toxins.

Robert Herron, PhD, Director of Research at the Institute of Science, Technology and Public Policy at Maharishi University of Management in Fairfield, Iowa, says that:

"Lipophilic (fat-loving, eg.- stored in fats) toxicants are generally considered to be among the most problematic environmental contaminants and many (but not all) of them have been banned in the U.S. for decades. Because of their fat-soluble nature and their long half-lives, they tend to accumulate in plants and animals and biomagnify up the food chain, increasing in humans with age. Previous studies show that these toxicants have been associated with hormone disruption, immune system suppression, reproductive disorders, several types of cancer, and other diseases." [16]

What's In *Your* Fridge?

Regarding soybeans, even John Robbins, author of The Food Revolution and an advocate of soy, acknowledges about soy that: "According to Monsanto's own tests, Roundup Ready soybeans contain 29 percent less of the brain nutrient choline, and 27 percent more trypsin inhibitor, the potential allergen that interferes with protein digestion, than normal soybeans. I find it fascinating that compared to regular soybeans, the genetically engineered beans have more of the very things that are problematic, and less of the very things that are beneficial. To my eyes, this is certainly another reason to eat organic foods whenever possible."

"It can be hard to find foods that don't contain soy flour, soy oil, lecithin (extracted from soy oil and used as an emulsifier in high-fat products), soy protein isolates and concentrates, textured vegetable protein (TVP), hydrolyzed vegetable protein (usually made from soy) or unidentified vegetable oils. Most of what is labeled 'vegetable oil' in the U.S. is actually soy oil, as are most margarines. Soy oil is the most widely used oil in the U.S., accounting for more than 75 percent of our total vegetable fats and oils intake. And most of our soy products are now genetically engineered."

Why are we eating so much soy protein? Because the chemical companies needed a way to get rid of all the waste created as a by-product of the soy oil industry:

Archer Daniels Midland (ADM) is among the largest processors of soybeans and soy products in the world. ADM along with Dow Chemical Company, DuPont and Monsanto support the industry trade associations United Soybean Board (USB) and Soyfoods Association of North America (SANA). These trade associations have lobbied hard and marketed fiercely to create an exponential increase in the consumption of soy products in recent years.[17] It's estimated that Monsanto seeds now account for 90 percent of the U.S. production of soybeans.[18] You'll see these same few names again and again when we talk about control of our food supply.

Of the pernicious lipid-loving organochlorine pesticides not yet banned in the US as of this writing, one of the worst is endosulfan. These are the countries which have banned it, as of 2008, and its status in those countries still using it:

World-wide regulatory status of endosulfan:

Bans: Countries that have banned endosulfan include Bahrain, Belize, Cambodia, Colombia, Cote d'Ivoire, Jordan, Kuwait, Malaysia, Norway, Oman, parts of the Philippines, Qatar, Saudi Arabia, Singapore, St Lucia, Sri Lanka, Sweden, Syria, and United Arab Emirates. In February 2008, Benin announced that endosulfan would be banned once existing stocks are used. Nine West African countries have recently banned the use of endosulfan in cotton—Senegal, Mauritania, Mali, Guinea Bissau, Burkina Faso, Tchad, Cap-Vert, Gambia, and Niger. Endosulfan is effectively banned in all the European Union countries. This brings the total of countries known or believed to have banned endosulfan to 57. It is also banned in the state of Kerala, India, as a result of severe adverse effects arising from aerial spraying of endosulfan on cashew plantations.

Reassessments: Brazil, Canada and the USA are reassessing endosulfan.[19] (In other words, still using it.)

Endosulfan is a highly toxic, bioaccumulative pesticide which that travels long distances and persists in the environment. Endosulfan is used on coffee, tea, cotton, vegetables, fruits. Among the many disorders it causes are early onset puberty in girls and delayed and stunted sexual maturity of boys. It has caused deaths, cerebral palsy, central nervous system disorders, cancers, and reproductive disorders.

Yet, even in the countries where it has been banned, the companies Dole and Del Monte have gotten exemptions to enable them to continue using it on products which are then shipped to this country for your children to eat.

Astonishingly, another omnipresent oil used by processed food companies in innumerable products is cottonseed oil. Cottonseed oil? Cotton is not considered a food product so cotton mega-farms are not even subject to the "stringent" regulations to which the EPA (Environmental Protection Agency) holds soy or other food crops. Read what the Organic Consumers Association (http://www.organicconsumers.org/) has uncovered about growing cotton:

What's In *Your* Fridge?

- [ ] Cotton uses more than twenty-five percent of all the insecticides in the world and 12% of all the pesticides. The US is the second largest grower. (China is first.)

- [ ] Cotton growers use 25% of all the pesticides used in the US. Yet cotton is farmed on only 3% of the world's farmland.

- [ ] The California EPA reported that only 15 chemicals accounted for 77% of the pesticides used on cotton from 1989 to 1998 and that these were some of the most toxic chemicals in the world. (California is one of the few states where farmers are required to provide pesticide use reports.)

- [ ] Cal EPA and US EPA analyses illustrate that seven of these fifteen most used cotton chemicals were probable cancer-causing pesticides, eight caused tumors and five caused mutations. Twelve of the top fifteen cotton pesticides in California caused birth defects, ten caused multiple birth defects, and thirteen were toxic or very toxic to fish or birds or both.

- [ ] Cotton fertilizers and pesticides have killed and injured millions of fish, birds, and other wildlife as well as countless thousands of rural residents.

- [ ] 75% of the cotton and cottonseed in the US is genetically modified.

- [ ] In the US we **eat** or **drink** more cotton products than we sleep on, wash with, or wear.

- [ ] Cottonseed accounts for about 60% of the harvest tonnage, gin trash (leaves, fibers and twigs) 5% to 20%, and cotton fiber only 30 to 35%.

- [ ] About 80% of all the cottonseed and almost all the gin trash go right into our milk. The other 20% of the cottonseed is made into oil, meal and cake and winds up in many different junk foods.

- [ ] An average of eight pounds of cottonseed is fed out to most dairy cows in the US every day.

- [ ] In addition to GMO cotton seed and gin trash, the cows are also fed GMO corn and soybeans. Many are also shot up with genetically modified bovine growth hormones. This makes milk one of the most toxically produced and genetically modified products. Since kids drink the bulk of the milk in the US, kids get the most poison as well the most exposure to genetically modified bacteria, viruses, hormones and antibodies."

Yet cottonseed oil, unregulated in terms of food restrictions, turns up in an astounding array of baked goods and other foods. These are just a few of the commonplace, known to be dangerous, components of the foods most of us eat everyday.

Another entire class of hazardous ingredients comes in the form of sugars. According to USDA data, in 2000, we ate an average of 31 teaspoons a day of various sweeteners. "Americans eat a pound of sugar every two-and-a-half days" says food historian Kathleen Curtin. In the 1700's each English person ate an average of about a pound of sugar per year.[20]

The consumption of high-fructose corn syrup (HFCS) climbed from *zero* in 1966 to 62.6 pounds per person in 2001.

Four companies control 85 percent of the $2.6 billion HFCS business— Archer Daniels Midland, Cargill, Staley Manufacturing Co. and CPC International.[21] Aspartame (NutraSweet) was originally made by Searle, a chemical company (and brought to market under extremely shady circumstances,[22]) and is now pushed by Monsanto. Saccharin was developed by Sherwin-Williams (think: paint) and is now owned by PMC Specialties Group, makers of a line of "Biocides" (literally, "killers of life") as well as pharmaceuticals, among other chemicals. Strangely, this includes a line of Saccharin just for animal feeds. (Apparently animals respond to sweet tastes just like we do, hence, like us, they can also be enticed to consume garbage disguised as food if it tastes sweet.) Saccharin therefore becomes another ingredient fed to cattle, swine, poultry. Even if you thought you were avoiding saccharin, you've been getting it in your meat. And around it goes.

Eating processed food is eating poison. But processed foods and meats are not the only dangers in our supermarkets.

There are also the residues of neurotoxins and petrochemicals we accept (on the counsel of the USDA) in our vegetables and fruits. Here is a small sampling of 10 common fruits and vegetables from the website

What's In *Your* Fridge?

Healthy Child, Healthy World:

Peaches

Peaches contain high residues of iprodione, classified as a probable human carcinogen by the Environmental Protection Agency (EPA) and methyl parathion, an endocrine disruptor and organophosphate (OP) insecticide. Methyl parathion has caused massive kills of bees and birds. According to Consumer Reports, single servings of peaches "consistently exceeded" EPA's safe daily limit for a 44-pound child.

Apples

Apples may contain methyl parathion. Both fresh apples and baby food applesauce can also contain chlorpyrifos, an OP which has caused large bird kills.

[Apple orchards are commonly sprayed with organophosphate pesticides, nerve agents that studies link to decreased intelligence and increased attention problems in children (Pediatrics, 2006, vol. 118, no. 6). "Apples appear regularly in the cafeteria of every North American school," says Ronnie Cummins, national director of the Organic Consumers Association." It's unbelievable they haven't made the switch."

According to EWG analysis of USDA and FDA data from 2000 and 2004, more than 93 percent of conventional apples tested positive for pesticide residues. One out of every eight times a child under age 6 eats an apple, the group estimates, he exceeds the Environmental Protection Agency's reference dose for organophosphates.[23]]

Pears

Pears, both fresh and in baby food, can also come with methyl parathion, as well as the OP azinphos-methyl, which is toxic to freshwater fish, amphibians and bees.

Winter Squash

Dieldrin, a chlorinated, carcinogenic insecticide, exceeded the safe daily limit for a young child in two-thirds of positive samples. Another potent carcinogen, heptachlor, also showed up. DDT and its breakdown product, DDE, were detected in baby food squash.

Green Beans

Green Beans can contain acephate, methamidophos and dimethoate (three neurotoxic OPs), and endosulfan, an endocrine-disrupting insecticide, which showed up in baby food, too. Acephate disorients migrating birds, throwing them off course.

Grapes

U.S. grapes contain methyl parathion and methomyl, a carbamate insecticide listed as an endocrine disruptor; imports may contain dimethoate.

Strawberries

The enhanced red color of strawberries comes from the fungicide captan, a probable human carcinogen that can irritate skin and eyes, and is highly toxic to fish. While the lethal soil fumigant methyl bromide doesn't show up on the fruit, it has harmed California farm workers, and depletes the ozone layer.

Raspberries

Watch out for more than thorns! These berries can contain captan, iprodione and carbaryl, a suspected endocrine disruptor that has also been found in plum baby food

Spinach

Permethrin, a possible human carcinogen, and dimethoate dominate spinach's toxicity ratings, but CU notes that residue levels have been declining as U.S. farmers reduce use of these insecticides. DDT has been found in spinach, which leads all foods in exceeding safety tolerances.

Potatoes

Pesticide use on potatoes is growing, CU warns. They may contain dieldrin and methamidophos, and children eating potatoes risk getting a very high dose of aldicarb, CU says.[24]

If it wasn't enough that all these residues were a result of chemicals sprayed on our crops, if you wonder who thought of feeding road kill and the chem-soaked bodies of euthanized animals to our livestock, know that for decades we have also been spreading an unfathomable array of noxious chemicals on the soil of our farmland as fertilizer.

Diane Olson Rutter, staff writer for Catalyst Magazine, told readers in May 2003 what was reaching her community:

"A sickening flow of heavy metals, nerve gas residue, dioxin, PCBs, pesticides, industrial solvents, petroleum oils, and radioactive plutonium, americium, radium and strontium-90 makes its way from the Lowry Landfill Superfund site southeast of Denver, down 17 miles of pipe, and into the Denver Metro sewage treatment plant. There it joins the city's domestic and industrial waste, and comes out the other end as sludge, which is used to *fertilize wheat.*"

Wheat is only one of the countless food crops nationwide subjected to this abomination. These crops then take up the heavy metals and other toxins into their roots, stems, leaves, fruit, and seeds.

Shockingly, the EPA has blessed this practice with the moniker of "recycling" of these hazardous wastes, for which the companies involved –who would otherwise have had to pay hazardous waste disposal fees– instead actually received public grant monies for "educating the public" about their recycling programs![25] And then they made television commercials to tell you how "green" they were. They're laughing up their sleeves at our ignorance.

The EPA has repeatedly chosen to work hand-in-hand with industry to assure the continued flow of money into corporate and political pockets with complete disregard for the health and safety of American citizens or our food supply. An example of this foot dragging, revealed by Earthjustice, *earthjustice.com*, (whose compelling logo is: "Because the earth needs a good lawyer") :

November 16, 2006 Seattle, WA -- The Environmental Protection Agency (EPA) announced today it will phase out the use of a deadly pesticide, AZM, developed from World War I-era nerve toxins that poisons farmworkers and injures their children. During World War I, it was the oil industry that began to create the poison gases for the war. After the war their market began to wither until they realized a new market for the nerve gases as bug killers on the farm. Although not all farm poisons are now nerve gas related, the origins of the pesticide industry lay in WWI and are still based in the chemical-petroleum industry.

The phase out will take six years for the most widespread uses of the pesticide, which will continue to subject workers and their families to poisoning risks.

"This pesticide has put thousands of workers at risk of serious illness every year," said Erik Nicholson of the United Farm Workers of America. "The phase out is welcome, but it is inexcusable for EPA to allow this pesticide to continue poisoning workers for 6 more years."

The pesticide, azinphos-methyl (AZM, also known as guthion), is a highly neurotoxic organophosphate insecticide. Organophosphate insecticides attack the human brain and nervous system. In 2001, EPA found that AZM poses unacceptable risks to workers, but it allowed the pesticide to continue to be used for four more years because less toxic alternatives might cost a bit more to use.

"With safer alternatives already in widespread use, the EPA has betrayed the trust of the men, women, and children whose health it is duty bound to protect by allowing this extremely hazardous pesticide to remain in use for six more years," said Shelley Davis, attorney for the Farmworker Justice."

Red Herrings

And now –instead of cleaning up the trail of sewage and toxins that gives rise to weakened animals and carcinogenic crops in the US– in 2006 our government approved a spray-on virus to be used on food products. Yes, live viruses. They're supposed to eat bacteria, which we are led to believe are the real dangers in our food supply. Says Siri Nilsson of ABC News:

> The FDA has now approved a virus-cocktail spray that might prevent listeriosis. The spray, called LMP 102, is a mixture of six different special viruses called bacteriophages — viruses that infect only bacteria, not people, animals or plants.
>
> Even though these bacteriophages cannot infect people, are they safe?
>
> Not completely. Bacteriophages, like all viruses, contain protein. These proteins can cause allergic reactions, just like milk proteins cause milk allergies.
>
> The bacteriophages might also get into battle with the friendly bacteria in the digestive system, making it harder for the body to digest food.
>
> But that's a risk the FDA already takes by allowing the use of antibiotics on farms. (and we've seen how well that's working... -my note)   This is the first time that the FDA has regulated the use of bacteriophages as a food additive. [26]

You know... I once knew an old lady who swallowed a fly. She swallowed a spider to catch the fly...

As of April 2007, the same company was working on getting approval for their latest treat, a virus spray that specifically eats E. coli, a bacterium which has been the subject of a great deal of misunderstanding and bad press in the last several years.

What's In *Your* Fridge?

John Vazzana, president of Intralytix, said that his company's anti-E. coli spray "would not affect so-called good strains of E. coli in the human digestive tract because the phages in his product are highly specific to O157:H7."[27]

I guess Mr. Vazzana and his team have never heard of mutations. Someone should introduce them to the work of Luria and Delbruck, published more than sixty five years ago. This article:

(http://www.accessexcellence.org/RC/AB/BC/Bacterial_Mutations.html)

explains it nicely in simple, laymen's terms. An excerpt:

> It was well known that if a bacterial virus was added to a flask containing bacteria, the liquid in the flask would become clear, as if the virus had killed all the bacteria.
>
> However, with time, the flask would once again become cloudy as the bacterial population rebounded - now composed of virus-resistant bacteria.
>
> This happened even when all the bacteria in the flask were the clonal offspring of a single bacterium. Although such bacteria should have all been genetically identical, some of them were susceptible to the virus while others were resistant.

Luria and Delbruck, in 1943, went on to describe how mutations work—more pointedly, the mutation of bacteria exposed to viruses "highly specific" to them. So much for not affecting the "good E. coli" in our intestines.

Did you know that the "good" E. coli bacteria are actually responsible for providing nearly all the crucial vitamin K in our systems?

Hundreds of years ago we had no idea what caused disease. Diseases like the plague were thought to be the result of "God's anger" or "the devil's evil" unleashed on the masses. In time people came to believe that rats spread the plague and great efforts were made to eradicate rats.

Later, it was found that it was actually the fleas carried by the rats which brought disease, and much attention was given to trying to eradicate fleas.

And then we discovered that in fact the fleas carried something even smaller, bacteria, and it was bacteria that were making us ill...

And now we are beside ourselves trying to eradicate bacteria. Hand towels, socks and underwear arrive impregnated with anti-bacterial chemicals, dish soaps contain anti-bacterial agents, as do laundry soaps, hand creams, gels, towelettes, ...and yet all the bustle and exertion have ultimately been fruitless.

We still have rats, we still have fleas, and not only do we still have "bad" bacteria, but if we stop and consider the idea of trying to eradicate bacteria when our own bodies are made up of at least 90% foreign microbes, most notably bacteria, the thought of trying to destroy all them is laughably naïve, very much an act of shooting ourselves in the foot.

There's more.

The newest mind-boggling assaults on our food supply are in the form of nanoparticles. Nanotechnology can broadly be described as the manipulation of nanoparticles or nanomaterials— matter thousands of times smaller than the width of one hair. Even as small as one molecule— far, far smaller than a virus. In terms of scale, think of prions, the infectious agents responsible for Mad Cow disease. (Whose ability to do damage is, at least in part, a direct result of their small size.) These materials have been quietly, almost surreptitiously, introduced into our foods within the last three years or so, typically for the purpose of –you guessed it– creating a longer shelf life in products.

They are now surprisingly widely used in packaging, clothing, electronics, manufacturing and cosmetics. Billions are being spent on ways to incorporate these materials into our lives. Food companies like Unilever, Kraft, Cadbury Schweppes, HJ Heinz, Altria Group (formerly Philip Morris Companies), Hershey Foods, and Nestlé are already involved. Drug companies like Glaxo-SmithKline are making nano-vaccines.

What's In *Your* Fridge?

Agriculture

Single molecule detection to determine enzyme/ substrate interactions

Nanocapsules for delivery of pesticides, fertilizers and other agrichemicals more efficiently
Delivery of growth hormones in a controlled fashion

Nanosensors for monitoring soil conditions and crop growth

Nanochips for identity preservation and tracking

Nanosensors for detection of animal and plant pathogens

Nanocapsules to deliver vaccines

Nanoparticles to deliver DNA to plants (targeted genetic engineering)

Food Processing

Nanocapsules to improve bioavailability of neutraceuticals in standard ingredients such as cooking oils

Nanoencapsulated flavor enhancers

Nanotubes and nanoparticles as gelation and viscosifying agents

Nanocapsule infusion of plant based steroids to replace a meat's cholesterol

Nanoparticles to selectively bind and remove chemicals or pathogens from food

Nanoemulsions and particles for better availability and dispersion of nutrients

Food Packaging

Antibodies attached to florescent nanoparticles to detect chemicals or foodborne pathogens

Biodegradable nanosensors for temperature, moisture and time monitoring
Nanoclays and nanoflims as barrier materials to prevent spoilage and prevent oxygen absorption

Electrochemical nanosensors to detect ethylene
Antimicrobial and antifungal surface coatings with nanoparticles (silver, zinc, magnesium)
Lighter, stronger and more heat-resistant films with silicate nanoparticles
Modified permeation behavior of foils

Supplements

Nanosize powders to increase absorption of nutrients

Cellulose nanocrystal composites as drug carrier
Nanoencapsulation of neutraceuticals for better absorption, better stability or targeted delivery

Nanocochleates (coiled nanoparticles) to deliver nutrients more efficiently to cells without affecting color or taste of food

Vitamin sprays dispersing active molecules into nanodroplets for better absorption

Examples for nanofood applications (Source: Nanowerk)
http://www.nanowerk.com/spotlight/spotid=1360.php

Nanoparticles are already on the market in the "clear" sunblocks you may be rubbing onto your toddler, in skin care and moisturizing products you rub into your own skin, in anti-bacterial socks, stain resistant clothes and dozens of other products. (And don't even think: "I've been doing it for three years already and nothing's happened." Cell damage may coalesce into disease a decade or more after the first confused twists of RNA begin to replicate—when your child is in high school and develops leukemia or when you, having used these products on your face, develop "unexplained" bone cancer in your 40's.)

Nanopesticides are already being prepared for our farm crops, though research shows bioaccumulation occurs in waterways. There are washing machines available which release billions of nano-sized silver ions into your clothing (to then rub off into your skin?), meaning more nanoparticles in the waterways. There are already clothes on the market with embedded nanoparticles, ready to come off in the wash. There are food wraps designed to be "smart" –to change color when food has gone bad– or which contain antibacterial nanomaterials to "protect" your food, but which may inadvertently leach those materials into your food.

Then there is the packaging which intentionally releases nano-preservatives into the food they are wrapped around. And there are nano products for use in food— an example is OilFresh, a product immersed into restaurant fryers so that they can use their oil for far longer than usual (yum!). Purportedly, a big goal for many of these companies is creating "healthier" ice cream or chocolate or fried foods. Is that really necessary?

So what's the big deal with nano foods? Well, as if there weren't enough adulterants and toxins already in our foods, now man-made nanoparticles can, in the way that prions have, enter our cells in ways and in places *never before possible.*

Here's how: In human cells, the average diameter of the nucleus typically varies from 11 to 22 micrometers.[28] A nanometer (nm) is 1,000 times smaller than one micrometer. In other words, it is ten to twenty thousand times smaller than the nucleus of the average cell. And the nucleus contains the bulk of the cell's DNA, the blueprint guiding its accurate reproduction.

Nuclear pores are the holes in the membrane surrounding the nucleus through which materials are able to pass, much like the pores in our skin. Nature designed these pores to be typically no more than 9nm wide in order to prevent most molecules from entering—because they would damage the nucleus, the DNA and/ or the cell, and thus damage the organ system the cell is in, and by extension the person who owns that organ system. You.

But here come nanoparticles in our vegetable oil, our M&Ms, our toothpaste, some no larger than *1* nm, certainly able to float through a 9nm pore and potentially wreak havoc wherever they go.

"Little nano-risk research is conducted by agencies that oversee health and environmental regulations."[29] says Robert F. Service, writing for *Science* magazine. The small amount of research that has been done on nanoparticle toxicity has shown it to be extremely dangerous.[30] The potential for future generations is truly frightening. We do know that these particles can cross the blood-brain barrier, as well as cross through the placenta. They can float freely through our bodies into our organs and into the deepest reaches of our cells. They could potentially wind up in our lungs by way of our clothing, in our brains by way of our lunch, in our children by way of their pregnant mother's moisturizer.

Do nanoparticles accumulate? We don't know. Do they interact with medical implants? We don't know. Will they harm your fetus or cause Alzheimer's? We don't know. Can they enter our gametocytes and be passed on to future generations? We don't know. Are they already in the marketplace? Yes.

We also know that scale can change the properties of many materials, so that for instance, gold can be made magnetic at nano scale and aluminum becomes explosive. In other words, even materials we thought we knew, we don't know at the nano level. And there's much, much more that we don't know at all.

Regulations? According to Barnaby J. Feder of the NY Times, FDA officials said in 2006 that "treating every new nanotechnology product that consumers swallow as a food additive might compromise the agency's mandate to foster innovation and might not be within its authority."[31]

Furthermore, on the FDA's own website, they state:

> FDA regulates only to the "claims" made by the product sponsor. If the manufacturer makes no nanotechnology claims regarding the manufacture or performance of the product, FDA may be unaware at the time that the product is in the review and approval process that nanotechnology is being employed.

But like so many recent food technologies, absolutely no

labeling is required to indicate that nanomaterials are in or on your food, so how would they know?

This was said, regarding the EPA's recent regulation (after public outcry) of one small facet of the nanomaterials industry, silver nanoparticles:

> Chemistry World has learned that manufacturers will not have to answer searching questions about toxic effects specific to the small size or shape of their silver particles; the real concern of those who want to regulate nanotechnology.
>
> Jim Jones, director of the EPA's Office of Pesticide Programs, confirmed that only standard protocols relating to the known aquatic toxicity of silver would be tested (for example, a product's levels of silver exposure). The extra 'nano' effects of any nanosilver product would not be tested for - nor did the EPA know how to do it.
>
> 'We haven't figured that out. No regulatory authority has figured that out,' Jones told Chemistry World.
>
> As David Berube, communications director of the International Council on Nanotechnology, commented to Chemistry World: 'If Samsung hadn't been so insistent on calling it nanosilver, this publicity would never have happened.'

The International Council on Nanotechnology, in the words of its director, has only one concern: negative publicity. If you don't know, they can get away with whatever they want.

The EPA, in a February 2007 White Paper*, states: "The EPA is actively participating in nanotechnology development."[32] Well then, it hardly seems that they will be the ones to regulate with our safety foremost in mind. In fact, the single, predominant fear of all nanoparticle manufacturers and regulating bodies? That consumers will find out.

In 2005 newspaper *USA Today* exclaimed enthusiastically that nanoparticles really are becoming "this generation's plastic."[33] As if that were a good thing. We're just now seeing the tip of the iceberg with respect to the ravages of PVCs: Dioxins and phthalates are irrefutably linked to numerous cancers, cirrhosis, endocrine problems. Bisphenol-A is showing up in all kinds of foods.[34]

How long will we eat and breathe and wear nanoparticles

before we find that they are seeping into the innermost depths of our cells and causing damage? Since they require no labeling, cannot be tasted, smelled or seen and the average medical facility is not equipped to recognize afflictions at a less-than-cellular level, I suspect it will be quite some time.

Look at all the autism spectrum disorders we have in society today, as just one example of something that was unheard of by the average person just 50 years ago. Something is happening to our offspring, something paralleling the explosion of pesticides, plastics and the industrialization of our food and our environment. We do not even have the technology to figure out what is going wrong.

Asbestos is commonly cited as an example of Western culture's reckless enthusiasm for a product which had not been well researched before being used with wild abandon and devastating consequences. Thalidomide is another. Nanotech is already on the same path.

(* A white paper is an article that states an organization's position or philosophy about a social, political, or other subject, or a not-too-detailed technical explanation of an architecture, framework, or product technology.)

How is it that we've gotten to a place where so many products that we find in our groceries, in convenience stores, in our fast food eateries, come labeled as food products if they have no nutritive qualities and in fact are detrimental to us? How is it that we've come to knowingly and placidly accept the routine daily ingestion of substances which are harmful?

Most of us by now have become hardened to the warnings about various dangerous chemicals and adulterants in food. They are in the news virtually every day. Meat recalls have become commonplace. There was a time when eggnog made with real eggs (usually from the hens out back) was a standard and delightful holiday drink, a time when body builders touted the benefits of slurping raw eggs for protein building; now fears of salmonella, listeriosis, E.coli run rampant.

Few would consider eating a raw commercial egg these days. Likewise, the dangers of polluted seafood are recited regularly by chipper newscasters before assuring us that everything is fine. Rare steak is virtually a thing of the past —we're warned in dire tones to cook meat all the way through— as if (and they want us to believe this), as if it was through the homemaker's wrongdoing that someone might get sick from the putrid filth that is commercial meat.

We no longer trust our food. How could we? With all the warnings and the constant contradictions, we're left in perpetual confusion. It's a state of mind so all-pervasive that we've become fatalistic about it. We eat within the background noise of dread; the little voice that says "this is probably bad for me" chatters incessantly like a faint radio station in the back of our minds. So we tune it out indiscriminately. We are allowing ourselves to be fooled.

"Baywatch" Food

A long history of one-upmanship by marketers for supermarkets, mega-farms, and science labs has resulted in our shelves being stocked with what I call "Baywatch Food." These are the unpackaged goods which appear to be real foods as grandma knew them: meats, fruits, vegetables, healthy and wholesome. Yet, they are strangely... better than wholesome. They are perfect. With the proliferation of supermarkets in our society after WWII, competition intensified between chains. Each grower, each chain of vendors called out to the consumer to notice its own larger, glossier, redder (or greener, or yellower) vegetables, its pinker meats. Each emphatically boasted its "buff"-er comestibles like a marathoner promotes his running shoe. Each brand claimed title to a fresher, more flawless product.

By the 1950's, the early supermarket consumer, accustomed to tweaking tomatoes, checking apples for bruises, found to his or her delight that they could buy tomatoes which felt perfectly ripe and exhibited uniform redness. Apples were without blemish, as were fruit and vegetables of all kinds. Not a single insect bite. No brown spots, skins of a magnificently uniform color and shine. And size? Over time, within this author's lifetime, lemons became the size of oranges, oranges the size of grapefruits, grapefruits the size of cantaloupes, cantaloupes the size of small watermelons. Apples became as large as softballs; a banana- a meal for two. Beef cuts were unfailingly, endlessly fresh. Chickens became the size of small turkeys. Turkeys have become a meal for ten.

Few people at that time considered the detrimental effects of the pesticides which kept those foods unblemished, now widely known. No one would have guessed then that the very fertilizers which provided for all that bounty were extracting a toll from each item grown as well. Everything simply grew larger and better in just the way we desired: the tangible realization of our imagined ideal. Each apple, each tomato fulfilled our innate human yearning for symmetry and visual perfection.

Today perusing produce at the supermarket is comparable to watching an episode of the late 1980's television show Baywatch, notorious for its actors who were "ripped", buff, augmented, insipid and vacuous. An apparently perfect product, yet empty. Our fruits, meats, vegetables, and other edibles, not only harboring a witch's cauldron of chemical residues, have become eye-candy: fake, devoid of life, and devoid of nutrition. Said Chuck Benbrook, chief scientist for the Organic Center:

> "The problem is that until recently, no one ever checked to see what was happening to the nutritional value of these much larger tomatoes, bigger grapefruit and the rest of the crops.

> Now we're in trouble. Not just the U.S. but almost every Western country that is using improved growing methods."

> Agriculture's "almost single-minded focus on increasing yields created a blind spot" in nutritional content, said Brian Halweil, author of the Organic Center's report, "Still No Free Lunch."

> "Almost more alarming, this decline has escaped the notice of scientists, government and consumers," wrote Halweil, a senior researcher at the Worldwatch Institute and a member of the Organic Center's scientific advisory board.

> The report said studies found:

> The more a tomato weighs, the lower its concentration of lycopene, a natural anti-cancer chemical that makes tomatoes red. There is also less vitamin C and beta carotene, a nutrient linked to vitamin A.

Milk from high-production dairy cows has lower concentrations of fat, protein and other nutrition-enhancing components than the milk from dairy operations of 20 years ago or more.

Sweet corn, potatoes and whole-wheat bread show double-digit declines in iron, zinc and calcium. The time span of the decline varies depending on the product studied but generally ranges from 20 to 100 years.

Over the years, improvements in seeds and plant stock not only grew larger plants but permitted them to be grown closer together and crop yields soared.

"Of course we're now capable of feeding more people, but what's happened is that unintentionally, the nutritional value of our food supply has been eroded," Benbrook said.

[http://seattlepi.nwsource.com/national/331421_bigfood13.html]

Having worked in food service, I have witnessed first hand the choices a mouse will make in a commercial kitchen. It will have scurried past the bags of brown sugar, past bags of white sugar, past bags of white flour and gone straight for the rolled oats. When the rolled oats are repackaged in sturdier containers, it finds the walnuts. [Yes, the mouse issue was resolved.]

What has happened to us that the human individual, an animal, a biological entity presumably striving to sustain its own life, has lost the ability to make the choice that will sustain its life?

Has it come to pass that we, as a species, are no longer as savvy as the average mouse?

The riches of the earth's bounty sustained humankind for tens of thousands of years without the "benefit" of science. The foods we need for our bodies to thrive are right under our noses, exquisitely indecipherable by science: a rolled oat, a mango, a chickpea –unable to be duplicated.

We humans know about as much about the intricacies of micronutrients, the synergies between plant chemicals, the complexities of our cells, and the workings of live soil as we do about outer space. It's all a lot of mystery and speculation. We basically haven't a clue. And yet we've blithely stripped most of what we ingest down to it's barest constituents and then have the hubris to add back the things we think we need.

We have done the same to our soil- by pumping three things into our ground (potassium, nitrogen, and phosphorus which we call fertilizers) we got more yield, more of any given crop, per acre. But these crops had fewer of ALL the other micronutrients the soil provides. The next year we did it again, but the soil was already depleted. The crops had even fewer of the micronutrients we need. The fertilizers weren't as effective, so we added more of the big three soil nutrients. Each time the plants showed signs of duress -yields were low- we'd add more fertilizers. On and on for sixty, seventy years. We were, in essence, strip-mining our farmland. We never looked to see what we were doing regarding levels of nutrients we didn't know existed- how could we? The problem is: we don't *know* what we don't yet know.

For decades we've been trying to add more and more back to our foods as we suddenly realize (each time a new discovery is made) the value of the components which have been missing, as illnesses in huge swathes of the population repeatedly reveal deficits in commercial food supply. But we can never duplicate nature. As a result, today we are mired in a plague of diet related diseases.

Bread is a good example. We strip the wheat kernel of its folate, among many other things, when we mill and refine and bleach it into white flour. [We also currently use alloxan, a known diabetes inducer, to bleach our flour. Alloxan is the drug of choice to induce diabetes in lab mice free of the disease.*35] Scientists then discover that lack of folate (the natural form of folic acid) in its mother's diet is definitively linked to high incidences of spina bifida and other neural tube defects in newborns. [Whole grains had been a substantial source of folate.] So the government adds folic acid, synthetic folate, to our bread supply.

At this point, currently everyone who eats conventional commercial breads is force fed folic acid. Is there a problem with this? Well, it now seems that the elderly, an increasingly large demographic, are particularly vulnerable to an excess of folic acid, which in various studies has been linked additionally to colo-rectal cancer and Alzheimer's disease.[36] It can also mask a deficiency of vitamin B12, resulting in pernicious anemia.

Folate is primarily found in green leafy vegetables (think: foliage) though whole grains are also a very good source. If people had access to and enthusiasm for healthy natural organic foods, high in quality nutrients of all kinds, many of these tragic diseases could have been avoided.

But because our mindset and our technology only allow us to deal with components in sterilized isolation, we drop isolated components into the vat, looking for change only where it is profitable. Ida Hoos, renowned US sociologist, wrote: "A kind of quantomania prevails in the assessment of technologies. What cannot be counted simply doesn't count, and so we systematically ignore large and important areas of concern."[37] While she was not referring to our food supply, our approach to agriculture and food science has been to treat it in exactly the same way.

We are unable to measure synergy so it doesn't count. We are missing the forest for the trees. It is an approach to biology born out of industry. Bass-ackwards.

Centuries have passed since Descartes' time. It is time we got past his outmoded mindset; man is *not* a machine. (Though ironically, we take far better care of our cars than we do our bodies.)

Where is our sense of self-preservation?

Governmental regulations, commercial food science laboratories and we, ourselves, are to blame. On the laboratory front, alimentary alchemy has advanced to such a degree that our mere tongue and rudimentary (compared to other animals) olfactory ability are quite unable to distinguish a synthetic from the real thing. Furthermore, we are now so accustomed to accepting as real the poorly constructed flavors of our youth –banana flavor, watermelon flavor, cherry flavor, as well as beef flavor, chicken flavor and others—that we have often lost all reference to the nuances of the real thing.

In this way, we often unwittingly fool ourselves. Most of us alive today in the United States are from generations that grew up on at least some foods that were adulterated, manipulated or downright counterfeit. Twinkies and Tang, Kool-Aid, frozen dinners, reconstituted potatoes, turkey "breast" (the blended, boneless, skinless amalgam of protein in plastic), Egg Beaters and Wonder Bread, margarine, fish sticks, chicken nuggets, the list goes on and on.

These things became our "comfort" foods in some small way by virtue of their being the things that we knew, the tastes and smells of our youth, the things that not only bring nostalgia but which have formed our expectations of what food should be.

Sixty years ago, Burl Ives sang an old folk song, *The Riddle Song*, with the line "How can there be a chicken that has no bone?" Sadly, today just such a product —a tasteless, boneless, skinless, white-ish blob of animal proteins injected with flavorizers, moisturizers and stabilizers and sealed in plastic— is what most people think of as chicken.

An acquaintance of mine is a truck driver. After a customary daily breakfast of biscuits and gravy at the morning truck stop, he complained that it was "no good." I don't eat that dish, but thought "What could make biscuits and gravy taste bad?" It's nothing but white flour in two different forms. I asked him, "What was bad about it?" He said, " It was cold and it was lumpy." Had he even tasted it, I wondered? Besides salt, what *is* the taste of truckstop biscuits and cream gravy? Pepper?

There was virtually no nutritional value in the commercial biscuits and gravy he had eaten. In its typical manifestation, it is almost nothing but a big ol' mess of bleached, refined, white flour. The biscuits also contain a rising agent —baking powder- salt, probably sugar (or possibly HFCS), powdered milk and water. The "cream" gravy is flour and water with powdered milk, probably sugars, and salt and pepper. (Each of these products undoubtedly has additional preservatives, stabilizers, etc...)

But this was a comfort food for him, possibly tied in to childhood memories, the satisfaction of a full belly, pride in his Southern culture, and his expectation was apparently not about taste, but a uniformity of texture in the gravy and for the product to be hot. Nothing more. [It should come as no surprise that this man had cancer, diabetes and emphysema, having spent his life indulging daily in that dish and similar comforts: 12 Mountain Dews a day and a ½ carton of cigarettes.]

We know that white flour is flour that has been stripped of all its nutrients in the refining process. The bran, the vitamin E, the antioxidants are refined out. This leaves nothing but starch. The same thing used in old-fashioned wallpaper paste. It has a much longer storage life than any other type of flour.

This idea of shelf-life being a desirable quality in our food has become one of the main themes of conventional foodstuff. Over and over again we read that one of the benefits to consumers that a new process or GE modification will provide is "longer shelf life." Think about that.

Deliberate deception is the standard of the day at our meat counters. Here food science has worked diligently to keep grocers from having expensive turnover of outdated product. Our red meats are bloated with injected brines— water to make an old dried piece of meat seem moist, and salt and other additives to act as binders to keep the water in the meat.

And because sickly, ill-fed cattle are where the meat came from in the first place, flavor enhancers are also deemed necessary. Then, because fresh meat becomes brown sitting on a shelf, cuts of meat are packaged in carbon monoxide and carbon dioxide so that they will appear fresh long after Mother Nature's own timeline. This gives the meat a longer shelf life.

Green unripe bananas are gassed to appear ripe when the they hit the aisles. Ultra High Temperature pasteurization keeps milk on the shelves for up to six months. Herbs, spices, vegetables, eggs, bacon, beef patties, pork, grains and more have been suffused with radiation before being put on the shelves, all to preserve shelf life.[38]

In fact, many people are now touting irradiation of (eventually) our entire food supply. The issue is not whether it makes the food radioactive, that is a red herring. By calling attention to and discussing endlessly the fact that the food becomes only negligibly radioactive, not more than often occurs in nature, the media, led by the industry, produces a reassuring blitz of information which makes it seem as if the dangers have been discussed and dismissed. In fact, the dangers have been side-stepped.

Besides sterilizing the product it is used on, thus removing all life-giving properties from it— vitamin and mineral content is decreased, as is amino acid and fatty acid content, and in addition new "unique radiolytic products" are created.[39] These are toxins including known carcinogens such as formaldehyde and naphthalene, among others. These now remain in the irradiated foods. As early as 1975 these changes were shown to create deleterious chromosomal abnormalities in a study of children who were fed irradiated foods.[40]

It is also important to realize that the use of irradiation to kill dangerous bacteria has already proven to have been misused, in documented cases of old, spoiled meat being sent back to the manufacturer, re-irradiated and then put back on the shelves. With the use of radiation it has become impossible to accurately judge the age of cuts of meat.

Other fears include filthy processing plants and unsanitary conditions being "disappeared" with the magic of irradiation. Only tracking records attest to origin and datedness of these products. Oh, but wait... the USDA, at the behest of Big Ag, has worked for years to dilute and distort both COOL (country of origin labeling) and the concept of irradiation itself which, since 2002, they have fought in many instances to rename as "pasteurization" and other innocuous-sounding, hackneyed, double-speak terms.[41]

Outside the realm of the food itself, there are the very real dangers of the increased dispersal of small but very powerful amounts of radioactive materials throughout the nation for the purpose of irradiation. This means more radioactive materials on our highways, and radioactive materials in additional locations throughout our communities. Rather than a dozen or more hazardous sites with large - and hopefully - secure and protected stockpiles of radioactive materials, we risk blanketing the nation with tiny amounts of dangerous radiation everywhere.

When you sit down to a meal, do you find yourself thinking "This tastes like crap, but that's ok with me because I know it had a really long shelf life?" I don't think so. In the end, are we, the consumer, supposed to be pleased that a product can sit on the supermarket shelves for an eternity without souring or spoiling? This is of benefit only to manufacturers and middlemen.

What it means for us is that any life force at all has been stripped out of the product. It has become, molecularly, an (almost) inanimate object. In the same way that the mouse will pass up the food-like substances which have been stripped of their essential nutrient value, bacteria will also bypass substances which contain nothing in the way of life-giving significance.

This is precisely why these treated products do not go bad— bacteria won't have anything to do with them. So are we also no longer as smart as the average bacterium?

Both in nature and in nurture, we have moved away from knowing, as our primitive ancestors did, what is actually good for us, what is spoiled and what is fresh, what is food. Sadly, the vibrancy and rich flavor of real food is something with which we are often no longer familiar. Once we re-learn how to taste, we will no longer consider debasing our bodies with sterile designer groceries.

We deserve better than food which tastes "only a little flat" or "kind of cardboard-y." And it's time we demanded it. Not of "the authorities," who we blame, criticize, and entreat as if they were surrogate parents and we were hapless children: of ourselves. We are the ones who are ultimately in charge of the food we eat. "They" are not going to provide you with the most beneficial products because it is not in "their" best interest.

They are interested in shelf life, larger size (higher yield per acre), uniformity, and the ability to withstand the rigors of shipping hundreds or thousands of miles, in marketability, in sales, and yes, they even have a vested interest in your illness.

The very same chemical companies that are defiling your food are producing catalogs of pharmaceuticals to treat you for the heart disease, depression, hyperactivity, cancers, and myriad other physical and mental illnesses that you will get from eating their food-like products, the decoys.

Chew this over:

"**Aventis**   Aventis "crop sciences" include herbicides, fungicides, pesticides and genetically engineered food. http://www.cropscience. aventis.com/products/products.htm

Aventis Pharma is the pharmaceutical division: http://www.aventis. com/main/0,1003,EN-XX-24770-37160--,FF.html

Monsanto   Monsanto is owned by Pharmacia. The Pharmacia Corporation was created through the merger of Pharmacia Upjohn with Monsanto Company and its G.D. Searle unit. Monsanto website: http://www.monsanto.com,

Pharmacia: http://www.pharmacia.com/About/Index.asp

BASF   BASF- fungicides, herbicides, pesticides: http://www.basf. de/en/produkte/gesundheit/pflanzen/products/

BASF   - pharmaceuticals: http://www.basf.de/en/produkte/ gesundheit/nahrung

Merck   Merck is known widely as a pharmaceutical company http://www.merck.com/ Merck Research Company; Applications to Register Pesticide: http://www.epa.gov/fedrgstr/EPA-PEST/1996/ July/Day-10/pr-796.html

Merck produces chemicals and precursors for pesticides and other neurotoxins. Merck Chemicals for Industrial Applications - Listed in alphabetical order: http://www.merck-ti.de/tabelle/cia_tabelle. htm "Our broad range of Chemicals for Industrial Applications is widely used in many fields of production within the chemical and technical industries." http://www.merck-ti.de/set_cia.html

Dow Chemical   Dow Chemical produces both toxic chemicals and pharmaceuticals.   http://www.dow.com/products_services/

index.html   Dow Pharmaceuticals: http://www.dowpharm.com/

Dow's pesticide products include the organophosphate pesticide Dursban (a/k/a Chlorpyrifos/a/k/a RAID a/k/a Lorsban and is found in about 800 other pesticide products). Dursban was to be phased out and banned from indoor, yard and garden use by 2004 because of what it does to the developing brain.

The EPA was going to allow Dursban to "continue to be sold until current stocks run out" but Dow has been scrambling to get this delayed. [*A quick Google shows that it is readily available to anyone as of December 2009. My note.*]

http://www.time.com/time/covers/1101020422/poisons.html

Dupont Chemical   Dupont Chemical recently sold a pharmaceutical division to Bristol Myers Squibb. Dupont makes pesticides and drugs: http://www.dupontpharma.com/

Here is a list of other chemicals and neurotoxins that they produce: http://www1.dupont.com/NASApp/dupontcom/jsp/products/products/productsMain.jsp

Bayer   Industrial chemicals, "crop protection" products, pharmaceuticals. http://www.bayer.com/en/index_en.php

Bayer pharmaceuticals: http://www.pharma.bayer.com/   It is interesting to note that the Bayer corporation was originally the I.G. Farben Company with deep ties to the Nazis during the 1920s and 30s. I.G. Farben produced the Zyklon-B gas which was used in the Nazi death camps."[42]

Poisons are being applied to our soil, are leaching into our water, are being sprayed on our food substances and being taken up by their root systems. Poisons are being fed to, brushed onto, injected into the animals we eat. Poisons are spewed into the air and dumped into the ocean.

Even if you avoid all the laboratory concocted, synthetic, and counterfeit products we are encouraged to ingest, poisons are in us. Even if you were to eat 100% organically, there is poison in your food.

Everyone alive today carries within her or his body at least 700 contaminants[43], known by the new term "body burden." Our rivers and reservoirs, our groundwaters are infused with petroleum distillates, PCBs, mercury and other chemicals. For more than 20 years the EPA has allowed the "recycling" of lead, cadmium, arsenic, uranium, plutonium, antibiotics and a host of other medical wastes and heavy metals into our farmland.

Real foods like apples and potatoes have become nutritionally all-but-empty facsimiles of their former selves— Baywatch Foods.

Supermarket or Big Box meats are carefully fabricated illusions of healthy fare. Packaged foods, convenience foods, concocted foods are decoys: imitations created to get us to settle for something cheaper than the real thing, at a higher profit margin for the creator. It is illegal in most states to purchase raw milk from your neighbor, or to process your own organically raised livestock and sell it to your neighbors.[44] "I'm not about to tell the cattlemen what they are going to feed their cows," Richard Raymond, the USDA's undersecretary for food safety (at the time of this writing), has said.[45] Yet the USDA knowingly allows meat contaminated with E. coli to be sold to you.[46]

And screaming at us from every medium are flashing ads, jingles, and exuberantly kaleidoscopic enticements to eat products which should not even legitimately be considered food. All this from the same corporations delighted to have you develop a lifetime dependence on their drugs aimed at diet-based diseases; diseases derived from their decoy food products.

It's enough to make your head spin. Countless studies have already shown unhealthy correlations between chemicals in our diet, the poor quality of our conventional food, the dangers of junk food and the multitude of modern illnesses that beset us, yet the public argument is still mired in a denial debate very similar to the one that the opponents of global warming managed to foment for years. Scientists bought by Big Pharma, lawyers, lobbyists, public relations people, all work in concert with the sole intent of confusing you, wearing you down, tricking and deceiving you. Well, "follow the money", as the saying goes.

Similarly, for decades the billion dollar tobacco industry fought tooth and nail to inject doubt, chicanery, and deception into the studies showing that smoking caused disease, while thousands died. The men and women whose wealth and lifestyle derived from the sale of tobacco tied up court cases, funded reports designed to distort scientific studies, and used every method at their considerable disposal to discredit those who tried to show the truth, even as their own family members sickened from and succumbed to the use of tobacco.[47] That same obfuscation and sleight of hand is being used today, honed to an ever greater subtlety by the pesticide/ pharmaceutical/ "food" companies.

There is no more powerful example of the real allegiance of our food protection agencies than in their unwillingness to track food products which have been adulterated. The FDA, the USDA, the EPA should have the long term health of the public, of you and me, as their number one priority, bar none. Instead, corporate interests dictate policy. It is their pocketbooks being protected.

Former commissioner of the FDA, Dr Herbert Ley, in testimony before a US Senate hearing, commented: "People think the FDA is protecting them. It isn't. What the FDA is doing and what the public thinks it's doing are as different as night and day."[48]

It seems an irony, under the circumstances, that it is a part of the Department of Health and Human Services. Curt Furberg, M.D., one of the physicians whose research brought Avandia into question, has said of the FDA that "safety is just not a high priority for them."[49]

In an era when scientific proof is called upon in every discipline to provide the supreme criteria by which a path or method or program is evaluated, it is significant and telling that these agencies refuse to track changes in our food supply which could provide valuable long term evidence of either their harm or of their biological inertness. Surveys show that the majority of the American public has clamored for the tracking of cloned food, of genetically modified food, of irradiated food. Yet currently the FDA is in the process of relaxing the already subtle labeling of irradiated foods and repeatedly refuses to consider labeling other methods of food adulteration.

We are understandably overwhelmed. We are tired, literally. Unquestionably you know someone who suffers from one of the myriad diseases of Western culture, of which fatigue is a major component: chronic fatigue, adrenal exhaustion, thyroid problems, Crohn's disease, fibromyalgia, lupus, asthma, GERD, gallstones, celiac disease, MS, IBS, diabetes, hypoglycemia, depression, migraines, cancers, hypertension. The list goes on and on and on. We suffer from an epidemic of fatigue. These diseases are all tied (though not exclusively- smoking and other lifestyle choices contribute) to the same three root causes: inferior diet, lack of physical activity, insufficient sleep. These three are twined together like the cords that make up a stout rope; the consequences of a deficit of one effecting the others.

If the rope represents our national health, we are fraying.

If you feel burned out by all the conflicting data, you are not alone. It's easy to feel cynical, resigned, submissive in the face of such a tsunami of disinformation. That's just what they want. Talk about complacent- many young people don't even realize that this isn't the way it has always been.

Then there's this conundrum: if certain vitamins, minerals, and antioxidants are known to improve intelligence levels in children, if proper diet is shown to play a role in reasoning, thinking, and problem solving, (and it has been) then what are we doing to the next generation's ability to save themselves? Are you really too tired to take a stand to fight for your health, your family, their future?

More and more people have had enough of feeling ill, tired, lied to and manipulated. More and more people are outraged and are taking it upon themselves to notice, to take action, to change. Like-minded people from all walks of life who have watched a child sicken from cancer or struggle to breathe from food allergies, who themselves may be exhausted or in pain, are finding the strength to stand together to put a stop to the desecration of our food supply.

And so a movement has begun.

It's time to stop being on the defense and work on our offense. Is it too much to ask to have at least some expectation that that which we purchase to eat is meant to offer real sustenance and not just a temporary sensation of fullness? That it is able to provide us with suppleness and strength of body and sharpness of mind? That at the very least it is free from things that will poison us? No, it is not too much to ask. It is what we should expect of our food. Lay down your fork and listen up:

Food is life. It is your life. We really are what we eat. What else could we be?

It's time for you to take a stand. It's going to take all of us to halt this fearsome "progress" and it's going to take sacrifice. To start, let's take a closer look at how the defilement of our food affects our self-image and perceptions.

CHAPTER 2

Your Weight is Bigger than You

In the long view, no nation is healthier than its children.
~ Harry S Truman

At the time of this writing, fully 74.1% of Americans are regarded as overweight by our medical standards.[1] Our obesity rate, around 15 percent from 1960 to 1980, skyrocketed to 31 percent in the last 25 years, according to USDA statistics. In the same period, the percentage of overweight children has tripled among kids in both the 2-to-5 and 12-to-19 age groups, according to the National Center for Health Statistics.[2] It is estimated that more than eight million Americans are morbidly obese.[3]

Contrary to what many people want to believe, recommended weights were not formulated around an ideal of 19 year old, 6' supermodels, but based on studies of past generations of average adults, spanning both a broad age and economic range. In the last two decades, despite all the focus on weight issues, the changes in fast food fare, the lawsuits, the lectures, why has the incidence of overweight more than doubled?

In 1940 in this country, only 7% of people were overweight.[4] Look at pictures of civic groups, home-maker's groups, Knights of Columbus or other similar lodge groups, high school graduation classes. If you're thinking that 1940 was a tumultuous time and that maybe Americans at that time were suffering between two World Wars and therefore it may not be representative, then pick another decade before 1970. Pick 1920 or 1960. Look for yourself. The truth is that in the early-to-mid decades of the 1900's, people still paid money just to *see* a five hundred pound woman. Nowadays, in many parts of the country it isn't unheard of for a five hundred man or woman to be standing in line in front of you at Walmart or sitting next to you on an airplane.

So let's dispel a few myths right away. Your ancestors were not fat. Your bones are not particularly large. You don't have bad genes. You don't have a fat-making viral infection. The average American eats

64 lbs. more meat, poultry, and fish a year than his or her counterpart in the 1950's. This is almost 50% more than 60 years ago.[5] We are correspondingly nearly twice as heavy, on average.

Everywhere from airlines to automobile manufacturers, to the rides at Disney's amusement parks, seats have had to be made larger to accommodate an average 15% weight gain in American adults in the last 45 years. News sources parade 1000 lb. men and women across our television screens several times a year.[6] Extra length has been added to seat belts and shoe laces. Extra sizes have been added to our manufactured clothing lines. (Though at the same time the actual size numbers, for women, have shifted lower to insulate us from that unpleasant reality, this is worth noting.) Even coffins have had to be made larger.

What is happening? This level of weight gain across the entire spectrum of Western civilization in such a stunningly short period of time is unprecedented in human history.

The problem is that WE have become the foie gras goose.

For those who may be unfamiliar with foie gras or its manufacture, let me explain. Foie gras is a pâté, a spread, made of goose livers. Geese, like all fowl, have been eaten for thousands of years. In the wild, prior to their yearly migrations, geese gorge themselves silly. It was found that the liver of such a goose was particularly tasty.

In centuries past, one might have whimsically thought of the goose as the little prince or princess of the barnyard. Always well fed and fat. In the final month of its life, though, it got just a little bit more. In emulation of their natural tendency to gluttony, some member of the farm would prepare a mash of corn and maybe oil and massage great quantities of it down the throat of each goose while the remaining geese queued up for their share. Geese fattened this way, even on artisan farms today*, clamor for their sweet, sweet corn even as they become rapidly obese and their livers grow fatty and ineffectual.

* On a modern factory farm a goose fares no better than a Tyson chicken. It lives in a wire cage barely larger than its body and force fed ad nauseam by machine through a tube.

Your Weight is Bigger than You

And what are we but the foie gras goose of the giant chemical industries? In the sixty years since the chemical, munitions and oil companies exploded from wartime concerns to become the civilian petroleum/pharmaceutical/pesticide industries, all interrelated and interwoven, Americans have been living like the fat little princes of the barnyard, growing wealthier, pudgier, and clamoring for ever more of whatever it was that was being offered. Ironically, just like the foie gras goose, much of that turned out to be corn in infinite permutations.

Now we're starting to get a little nervous. Our livers have grown fatty and are beginning to fail. We're out of breath and it's hard to waddle away. We're starting to think that maybe we don't want anymore. Yet what do we get but more... more pills, more diet drinks, more "super weight loss" foods, more mood altering chemicals to calm us in our panic, more sage advice and surgeries from medical authorities tied to the strings of Big Pharma, more wisdom from nutrition experts weaned at the university-teats of the chemical industries, and ever more modifications of that same sweet corn.

It's hard to feel like these products are not being forced down our throats— it's difficult to find anywhere in our lives where there is not an advertisement of some kind, nudging us to eat to drink to buy. If we are not actually the foie gras goose, it certainly seems like someone thinks we are.

Food (products) come at us from every direction. Even in what are considered rural areas, one can rarely travel more than five miles without encountering a convenience store selling almost nothing but chips, candy, pastries, numerous indistinguishable deep-fried things and soft drinks.

Fast food restaurants guide our travels like mile markers. Every thirty miles or less in most parts of the country, a McDonalds, a Waffle House, a Denny's; Big Boy, Burger King, KFC, Long John Silvers, Pizza Hut and dozens more capture our attention with bright colors and million dollar advertising campaigns intricately designed to manipulate our primitive impulses.

Billion dollar Agri-Pharm-Chemical companies have found it lucrative to feed manure, plastic and other unfathomables to animals, then pump them full of enough antibiotics and drugs to keep them barely standing; alive just until the payment for their sale clears at the bank, one might say. (Did you know that cattle which used to reach maturity at 4-5 *years* now reach maturity at 12-16 *months*?! And we wonder why our daughters are maturing earlier!) They spread heavy metals and sewage sludge on our farm soil, and grow our vegetables and grains in it with the aid of megatons of chemicals. And the real money is in creating concoctions in the lab which have very little to do with meat or grain or vegetables.

The point, as noted in chapter one, is that those *same* companies fattening livestock are the ones feeding *us*.[7] And providing *our* drugs. It appears that they'd like nothing more than to find a way to feed us manure and plastic directly, and much of what they sell us is, at least metaphorically, exactly that.

So what do we do about it? To approach this problem, we have to address several issues. One is to recognize the problem. You'd think that with all the media attention about obesity, health and diet, we'd have a clue that something isn't right. This isn't necessarily the case.

Food, weight, what to eat, what not to eat; we're awash in diet plans and books and programs, diet pills, diet patches, advice and suggestions of surgeries large and small. These familiar currently popular diets are the tip of the iceberg:

The 3 Day Diet	The Maker's Diet
The Atkins Diet	The Mediterranean Diet
The Candida Diet	The Raw Food Diet
The Cookie Diet	The Sonoma Diet
The Diabetic Diet	The Shapeworks Diet
The Engine 2 Diet	The Slim Fast Diet
The Glycemic Impact Diet	The South Beach Diet
The Grapefruit Diet	Weight Watchers
The Low Carb Diet	The Zone Diet

Your Weight is Bigger than You

We hear almost daily about some facet of health on the news. Some television stations have made a health feature a regular part of their programming. Most newspapers have a health section. Most magazines regularly run health columns, some are entirely about our health from one perspective or another. We hear about meat recalls, about food-supply related disease outbreaks, about food bills and farm bills before Congress. Scientists warn us, doctors exhort us, "experts" try to lure us to their latest cure.

It is an irony that we tend to associate the word "epidemic" with the poorer parts of the world and think of ourselves as strong, active, healthy, well-nourished. It simply isn't true. A 2002 study in the Journal of the American Medical Association revealed that at least 81% of Americans take some form of medication weekly.[8] Yet many people honestly still don't think there's a problem.

One headline claims: "Overweight but unconcerned; chubby, tubby, portly, stout: Americans may be more at home with a little extra padding, or so, these days." [9]   As Emily, a blog commenter, explains, "Plus size is average, plain and simple. Few people are skinny anymore. I don't see how saying "I'm average size" is a misperception when it *is* the average size." [10]

And it's true. The average size has broadened tremendously, and there are many people who, like Emily, think that we should simply accept that this is the new norm. What is troublesome about this is that with that extra weight comes a litany of health problems which that commenter and others like her are also accepting: limited range of motion, limited stamina, shortness of breath, knee pain, heartburn, gas, indigestion, acid-reflux,— surprisingly, we have also begun to accept these as *normal* even in people in their twenties or teens or younger.

Human nature is quirky. On the one hand we are decidedly a youth oriented society, billions of dollars are spent by people trying to retain the appearance of youth. At the same time, in small groups of friends or co-workers, we seem to like to boast about our incipient infirmities –the bad knee, the fatigue, the "can't lift (or walk or bend) as much as I used to", perhaps as a way of affirming our maturity, our adulthood, our seniority, our world-weariness even in our twenties or thirties.

So when we notice that we have acid-reflux, we find ourselves thinking "well, I'm getting older." A quick scan of the media serves to convince us that indeed, everyone suffers from reflux. We're shown slender young people after normal everyday events reaching for antacids. Worse yet, we see Jane or Joe Thirty-Year-Old grimacing at the thought of the spicy pizza or rich ice cream in front of them- and then taking a pill and eating it anyway!

We have come to accept a feeling of illness as a normal part of eating. Here is your body, obviously sending you a signal— saying *please, please, don't eat that.* And someone (the marketer) is trying to convey the message— "go ahead, eat it... heh, heh, heh... we can fool your body with this little pill."

I can't help but think of the little devil image that used to be shown sitting on someone's shoulder tempting them towards wrongdoing. That little devil has become an iconic gag, a throwback to a time of quaint simplicity. We like to think of ourselves as being able to "handle" temptations- we're edgier, savvier, worldly-wise, jaded. [Of course, every generation in recorded time thinks it's more worldly-wise than the previous one.] The difference is that Westerners today are encouraged (by marketers) to indulge in all life's temptations, which, as it happens, they will sell you. What we somehow don't see is the toll it is taking.

In just one example: there are dozens of over-the-counter antacids available in countless formulations—liquid, gels caps, granules, tablets, chewable tablets, fruity flavored, mint-y flavored. Alka-Seltzer, Maalox, Mylanta, Tums, Pepto-Bismol, Rolaids, Milk of Magnesia, Pepcid, Di-Gel, Caltrate; there are even bubble gum antacids targeted just for children, and nobody thinks this is weird??

In another example of placid acceptance of pharmaceuticals, Dr. Margaret Adamek tells us "Eighty percent of amphetamine prescriptions are written for children—and administration of amphetamines to children has risen 3,000 percent in the last ten years." [11]

A child who needs to take an antacid after eating is not a normal, healthy child! A twenty or thirty-something who needs to take antacids on a consistent basis is not normal. Even older people should not have to take a pill before or after eating, just to survive what they are ingesting. Chronic indigestion, flatulence, reflux, constipation, is not normal.

Doctors commonly suggest that we diet while prescribing a list of pills. We're bombarded with the message that it is the norm to suffer from heartburn and indigestion. Everyone seems to take some kind of medication. And so we believe that "this is how it is." We fail to realize that our state of illness is not the natural human condition.

"According to the Food Allergy & Anaphylaxis Network (FAAN) school nurses nationwide are reporting an increase in students with food allergies, and safety precautions should be taken to protect food-allergic students from reactions."[12] So, rather than wondering why our bodies and those of our children are disintegrating before our eyes, we outlaw peanut butter and jelly sandwiches in schools! And nobody thinks this is weird?

Over and over I've been astounded by people claiming a state of health when plain common sense pointed to the contrary. I once had a neighbor in her 30's who, at no more than 5'3" weighed over 300 lbs., and who insisted with vehemence that she was healthy- because she "wasn't sick!" She couldn't climb a flight of stairs without resting, but that was "just her weight" and not anything "wrong" with her. Somehow in her mind, other than as pertained to her appearance, her weight was not considered something manifestly, inherently wrong with her body. Fifteen years later at the age of 50, she was dead of sudden heart failure.

A co-worker of 32 or so was told by his physician that he was obese. He was not quite 5'7" and over 220 lbs. He was positively insulted by the suggestion and repeated the story to each of us for days.

"I'm solid" he insisted, "I'm just built this way." At the same time, he acknowledged that he'd first been admitted to a hospital emergency room for severe heart trouble when he was just 28. We are refusing to recognize the reality staring us in the face.

Overweight and obesity affects people in all economic strata, all races, all ages, urban, suburban and rural; it has swept through the Western world. It has health ramifications, economic ramifications, personal-satisfaction-with-life ramifications, emotional ramifications and hands down, all of these ramifications are negative.

If you're male, maybe you feel a certain pride in being a "big" guy. You like fast food and a few beers, you're never going to be one of those lettuce eaters. Maybe you just feel you're settling down and eating better since you got married. You're doctor has told you that you fall into the obese category and you just scoff. Look at all those other guys, they're fatter than you. Or maybe you've always been heavy and accept, like my co-worker, that this is "just the way you are."

Or maybe, male or female, you put on a few pounds because your job requires you to eat out, and in some way that weight is a part of your success, your hard work. You appreciate good restaurants and you can afford them. Or maybe you're not making the money you should be making and eating something you like, some treat, is your only reward.

Many women want to lose weight to fit a certain cultural expectation in appearance. But really, most of the time, you know... you look in the mirror and find that, ok, you're a little overweight, but it's not all that bad. Maybe you've learned to look at the bright side and note that you have nice lips, smooth skin, or great hair. Maybe you've accepted a Reuben-esque figure and feel it's just gotten a little out of control. Maybe you've always been heavy and you, too, accept that this is just the way you are.

So, what it boils down to is that, well, we want to look good, but it's hard, and complicated, and good becomes "good enough" and you know that your beauty is inner beauty, or your pride is in what you do or earn and looking svelte isn't all that important to you. That's ok. Really. It's good to feel comfortable with how you look.

The problem is that we shouldn't ever approach eating in terms of how we look. Yes, eating too much or the wrong things will make us fat, but that should not even be the issue. We have to think of food differently. How you look is fine. The question is: how do you feel? Eating as body image is a hall-of-mirrors approach to food. It reflects the issue back on itself in a convoluted charade that never ends. It misses the point.

This then, is the paradox. While overweight may indeed be the condition of the average person; obesity and gastrointestinal disturbances and lethargy may have become the norm, but that does not make them *normal* in the Merriam-Webster sense of "occurring naturally." The problem with Emily's deduction, above, is that it is a dangerous fallacy of logic: exactly the kind of thinking that marketers want you to come up with. Consider this: if 70% of a community suffers from some kind of cancer, do we simply say "oh, well, it's normal to have that cancer"? Of course not. It's normal to be healthy.

It's normal to be free from pain, free from autoimmune diseases, free from allergies, to be able to breathe without asthma, to be able to eat without distress. We are encouraged by medical professionals to consume pharmaceuticals for relief of symptoms. These symptoms are our body's way of crying out for attention. And our response is to simply stifle its voice.

It is imperative that we stop in our tracks, right now, and take a cold hard look at our behavior. *Eating is making us miserable.*

You shouldn't have to control your diet in order to be healthy. This is how we evolved: our body's messages told us whether a food was good to eat or not. Your body, in its primal, feral state, wants healthy food above all. Why is it craving anything else?

Something isn't right. The first step is realization. If you and everyone around you are suffering from chronic discomfort- colds, allergies, intestinal problems, aches, fatigue- even if they seem minor, even if it appears that everyone has these things, know this: something is wrong.

We're told how to eat from a thousand different sources. There are health foods and health programs, newsletters and authorities of all kinds, suggesting, cajoling, admonishing, and many people are trying, really trying to "be good." We spend almost $50 billion on weight loss programs in America.[13] As Marion Nestle says in her excellent book *What to Eat*, "for many people, food feels nothing at all like a source of pleasure; it feels more like a minefield." Why isn't all of this helpful advice "taking?" Because something is missing.

To be in pain is not natural. To feel bloated after eating is not normal, even if it is common. To feel tired when climbing a flight of stairs at the age of 35 or 45 or even 55 is not an inevitable fact of life. What has happened to the human species that we cannot tell that we are not well? This seems to be an epidemic, not just of obesity, but of inattention. We are experiencing a loss of direction, a numbness about ourselves, a culture-wide disconnect from our bodies.

It is important to grasp the fact that this is a cultural issue. And it is not just an American phenomenon, although we are leading the fat pack. There is an epidemic of complacency and resignation which seems to follow what has been called "the Western diet" like a shadow. But why? The Western diet is exemplified by processed foods, junk foods and fast foods with a high sodium, sugar and saturated fat content and a low nutrient density.

It has been linked to metabolic syndrome: a collection of risk factors for heart problems, stroke, colon cancer and type 2 diabetes among other things. And it is true that illness can lead to exhaustion and exhaustion can lead to resignation. But the Western diet is our cultural touchstone, a measure of America's success in providing food for all, abundant and cheap. It is who we are. And it seems to be what we want, isn't it? We're certainly told that all the time— despite clear evidence that it is killing us.

Resignation, complacency, even seeming to have blinders to

the changes in our world in recent decades is understood when one realizes that obesity has become, in many ways, the medium in which we now live. Even thin people are submerged in the environment of obesity: the shift in the size-names of women's clothing, the scarcity of smaller sizes in men's clothing, our style of clothes— oversized, bulky tops, baggy pants, untucked shirts, open laces, larger bucket seats in autos and trucks, seat belt extenders, roomier recliners, king-sized beds with firmer mattresses, fitness centers in every strip mall, our culture's incessant focus on calories; everywhere you look our society has adapted to the new obesity. It's all-pervasive.

Is it also possible that the same foods and habits which have made us sluggish, weary and out of breath have also made our minds a foggy jumble of short-circuited exhaustion? If so, is transformation hopeless? No. This does not mean that it is out of your control, quite the contrary.

Frequently when we struggle it is easy to believe we are the only ones dealing with a particular burden. Although we are bombarded with media debating weight and diet and statistics ad nauseam, people often feel as if they are alone in that moment of will-I-or-won't-I eat this "forbidden fruit." We tend to believe we are dealing with a personal problem and this brings feelings of inadequacy and a stigma of shame or sometimes a sense of defiance. It feels personal. It's not. In truth, your weight is our society's issue.

Unlike an issue which is your "fault", this is a condition that is being foisted on you. This is not about willpower. It's not that you've been "bad." It means that there are things which you may not have considered –or of which you may not even be aware– that have influenced and affected you and your family as well as your neighbors, your community and the rest of the nation. This is about you being scammed.

The Monkey House

You are being manipulated. Every aspect of human behavior has been studied over the last 60 years as never before in history. Not only our innate preferences like that for sugar, but our habits, our levels of tolerance, our weaknesses, our goals, our desires and every other conceivable facet of our lives. And you'd better believe those studies are being used to lure you to buy, to covet, to yearn.

Marion Nestle says of Vance Packard's book *The Hidden Persuaders*, "His most shocking revelation? Corporations were hiring social scientists to study unconscious human emotions, not for the good of humanity but to help companies manipulate people into buying products." His book was written more than half a century ago. The ability to study and track our behavior has reached levels Packard could not have conceived. And the tracking of behavior is for the sole purpose of attempting to orchestrate it.

In *Fast Food Nation*, Eric Schlosser reveals that "McDonald's used helicopters to help figure out how suburbs were growing, looking for cheap land along new highways and roads. The company sought places where lots of cars would drive past and children would live nearby. During the 1980s McDonald's became one of the world's largest purchasers of satellite photographs taken from outer space, using them to get an even better view of local neighborhoods."

"Soon, he tells us, "other companies started buying satellite photographs, and a technology that was originally invented to help the US military spy on its enemies became one more tool to help fast-food chains sell more hamburgers. Scientists at the Barcelona Institute of Technology are now using equipment to study the magnetic activity of people's brains as they watch commercials. When people feel strongly about a brand, it sets off a response in a specific part of their brain." What they are calling "Neuromarketing" is being used to "create loyal customers".

Colors on labels, background music, aromas, lighting, the temperature of the store, the fact that grocery store aisles have become one-way labyrinths forcing you past items you didn't come for and don't want; every detail has been meticulously assembled to coerce you to purchase from your gut, as it were; impulsively, unconsciously.

Who among us doesn't end up coming home from the grocery store with things we didn't intend to buy?

Aren't you tired of feeling like a little rat in a maze when you do your shopping? Don't you wish the interminable aisles had breaks so that you could cut through once you'd gotten what you needed? Don't you wish you could just enter the store from the middle instead of having to walk to the far end of the parking lot to the entrance so that you're placed in front of what they want you to see? And that you could walk right in to the aisle you need, look each way to find what you came for and then get it and be done?

If you came in for a sandwich, doesn't it sometimes irk you that you have to walk 50 feet in the other direction past all the roped-off register lanes, through all the promotions, and then back again on the other side to get to the deli? That something like milk or butter which nearly everyone gets, is invariably all the way at the back of the store?

In fact, the placement of the stores themselves, the design of their parking lots, even the design of entire neighborhoods are meant to focus you on the convenience of purchasing. Many communities are designed in such a way that makes it very difficult to try to grow food, to have a little garden: not enough sun between the McMansions, not enough space, sometimes no soil at all.

We're told that this is what we want, but as anyone who's bought a home knows, most of us move into what is available- what the developers have developed. Or what is in fashion; what we're led to believe we deserve. Likewise, our cars: for decades our vehicles have been designed larger and larger not only to encourage us to flaunt our personal purchasing power, but to entice us to fill them with all the things we are continuously told we should have.

Who hasn't said, "Why did I buy that _____," (fried turnover/ new pair of shoes/ CD/ video game/ fill in your own favorite weakness) and honestly wondered, "what was I thinking?"

Just as livestock have been intensively studied in order that producers can tweak their speed of growth, so have humans been studied. In CAFOs (Confined Animal Feeding Operations, sometimes known as factory farms or industrial livestock operations) it is common to de-beak and de-claw and sometimes even de-toe chickens to keep them from pecking and scratching each other in a frenzy of constant jostling and pungent, furious overcrowding.

With cattle, horns are removed for the same dismaying conditions; with pigs tails are removed, often teeth are ground down as well. All of this to prevent the expression of the animal's rage, frustration and anxiety not just from the horribly congested situation, but from constantly feeling unwell.

People are easier. Convince them to take antacids, painkillers, NSAIDs, for the discomfort, then SSRIs (selective serotonin re-uptake inhibitors) and other antidepressants for the despair, frustration and anxiety.[14] We think that we can fool ourselves when we take the pills enabling us to eat things that are not good for us. We think that we are successfully fooling ourselves when we take more pills to then cover up the resulting malaise, the dis-ease, the aches.

"Blithely consuming low-fat foods full of carbohydrates is a prescription for portliness," says Walter Willett, chairman of the department of nutrition at the Harvard School of Public Health, adding that any farmer knows this. "If you pen up an animal and feed it grain, it will get fat. People are no different."[15]

Like the cattle who, at a mere 16 months of age, wobble woozily to the slaughterhouse, achy, flatulent and ill—but considered "well" in the eyes of commerce, we consider ourselves well if we are still able to go through the motions. But our bodies are not fooled or we would not be in the throes of an epidemic of antidepressant use. Our bodies are calling out for our attention. We are being encouraged to silence those signals.

Let's look at diabetes. Diabetes, which had a per-capita incidence of 0.0028% at the turn of the last century, had by 1933 zoomed 1,000% in the United States to become a disease seen by many doctors.[16] This was alarming at the time. Today, according to the American Diabetes

Association, there are 20.8 million children and adults in the United States, or 7% of the population who have diabetes. Another study in the Journal of the National Medical Association (August 2006) puts that number at 8.5%. That is an increase of 300,000 *percent* since the turn of the last century.

Type II diabetes is caused by too many carbs and too much sugar of any kind in the system. Very simply, sugars and carbohydrates are rapidly converted to glucose in our bodies. Insulin is produced to push glucose into the cells for storage. When the cells can't handle anymore glucose they just stop accepting it. Looked at from one perspective, the insulin appears to not be doing its job. This is insulin-resistant diabetes. Insulin is no longer working to push the glucose into the cells. We are told that this is a failure of the insulin.

Consider this: picture your cells as storage units, or as your garage and basement. There are only so many places you can store stuff. Sugars, like fructose and sucrose, and carbs like bread, French fries, etc, when broken down all become glucose, that is— they are individual items which can be grouped under one heading, the equivalent of, say, your various kitchen gadgets.

And let's say you have an obsession, ahem- *collection*, and continuously acquire kitchen gadgets (glucose). The glucose is converted to fat molecules in order to be stored (imagine that the kitchen gadgets are now boxed.) The movers (the insulin) are hired in order to place the boxes (fat molecules) into storage (the fat cells.) Eventually, the storage rooms are going to become full.

Now, imagine that the storage unit walls are made of rubber. You can't buy more storage units. The cells that you have are all that you get. BUT, being made of rubber, you can stuff them, and stuff them, and ...stuff them. They bulge. They distort. They become grossly misshapen. Your fat cells are bloated. Finally, no matter what, your movers are exhausted, nothing can be re-arranged any further, the things in the back can no longer be gotten to, not one more decorative geegaw can fit into the garage. The movers quit. The insulin cannot move anymore fat molecules into the cells. This *could* be seen as a failure of the insulin.[17] But do you blame the moving crew because you have too many things?

This is a fanciful but useful analogy in thinking about how our bodies become diseased. The overwhelming majority of our illnesses are things that might have been avoided through a lifetime of eating judiciously. Unfortunately, judiciousness would not be profitable for the pharmaceutical industry, the diet industry, the food science industries, the geegaw makers, or any other industry interested in having you buy more.

The problem is of course, more complicated. It is a fact that normal, healthy cells require vitamins, minerals and other nutrients to function as intended. It is also a fact, as I've stated, that science doesn't know yet exactly what levels and combinations and subtle synergistic interactions create ideal health from the exponential number of possibilities that exist. If we look to what nature provided us in earliest times, we find lots of fruit and vegetables, some grains, some meats, some dairy. Humans thrived for tens of thousands of years on those essentials with little more than cooking or fermentation to alter them.

Now we live in an environment where edibles are altered beyond recognition. In olden days we used our natural inborn senses for assessing the quality of a fruit or vegetable or meat. Does it look ok? Mold, bruising, discoloration? Does it smell ok? Acrid, putrid? Does it feel ok? Has it become slimy, hard, soft, weepy? And finally, what does it taste like? A tiny taste could often tell us if a familiar food was "off." Now we can't trust any of that. As corporate/ industrial food behemoths acquired the ability to manipulate things at a level undetectable by our senses, (genetic modification, nano-materials, countless methods of chemical preservation) our innate facilities have been stolen from us. They have been made obsolete.

It looks good? Turns out that is a plastic apple. It smells fresh? That scent was created in a lab. Think about the fact that there is an entire realm of food science dedicated to developing "mouth feel." It tastes good? You can't use that as a criteria as to whether it is good for you: Can you judge how GM corn is affecting you at the cellular level? The argument that "if you can't tell, then it's not affecting you" is either specious or naïve.

What Are You Craving?

Nutrient imbalances from eating altered, depleted or fabricated food products create cravings because the non-food or nutrient deficient foods may interfere with nutrient absorption and create cellular deficiencies.[18] Cravings can even be caused by eating real foods, but in a way which constitutes an unbalanced diet. Many people who suffer from obesity have experienced the cravings caused by a diet wherein the sugars or carbohydrates far outnumber the other nutrients— a temporarily sated feeling followed shortly by the overwhelming desire for more carbs or sweets. Similarly, an alcoholic may interpret a sugar craving as a craving for more alcohol. In each case, the body doesn't really want more sugar or more alcohol, it wants nutrients, but we are distressingly unskilled in interpreting our bodies needs when confronted with abundance, with readily available alcohol and decoy food products in a society which sends a message that self-indulgence is our highest value.

When some pregnant women crave non-food substances, it is called pica and is often suspected of being related to iron deficiency. Children, usually in poverty conditions where they are not getting adequate quantities of food, also develop pica and are known to eat all kinds of items in order to satisfy a hunger for the micronutrients they are not receiving.

Craving is well known in the ranching community. Veal is the meat of very young calves denied iron. The animal is deliberately given a diet without iron to keep its flesh pale for the veal consumer. The tiny calf is denied bedding because it would eat it for the minute amount of iron in the straw. It is kept in a stall without iron fixtures because it would lick them to get iron, and it is denied the ability to turn around because it would lick its own urine to obtain iron if it could—less than

16 weeks old,[19] it knows instinctively what it needs and desperately tries to get it. Is this what decoy-foods are now doing to all of us, creating malnutrition in people of appropriate (or greater) weight? We are a nation craving.

This same craving by our cells for the raw materials they need to perform manifests itself in a multitude of ways that we do not recognize as imbalance until the crisis becomes a huge booming collapse of an organ or system. The cells are not getting enough of what they need, but let's face it, cells have a limited repertoire. They can't send an email or leave a note on the fridge if they are not being fed. They beseech us in their own way but our bodies are so dysfunctional that we don't give credence to the symptoms. We ignore them.

All the myriad warnings we experience— gastrointestinal illnesses, fatigue, the breakdown of organs (gallbladder, thyroid, pancreas, heart, liver, to name a few), all the symptoms associated with "Syndrome X" (a constellation of health problems related to insulin resistance), the astounding array of autoimmune diseases in today's society, all these are the cries of our cells, their keening and lamentation... until finally, like an ill-tended house plant, they die. You may look at the shriveled little ficus in the corner and think, "it happened just like *that!*" But it didn't.

What we eat impacts our ability to think, our energy level, our tolerance for noises and stresses, our perception of and interpretation of events, our emotional grip on our lives. It is important that we understand that the foods we eat are leaving us craving at a very basic level. Sometimes we interpret those cravings as desire for more food when we know very well that we just ate and shouldn't be hungry. Other times it is more insidious. We crave *something...*

We feel uneasy, agitated, unfocused. Maybe a new diet would do the trick or a new hairstyle, maybe what we need is a new job or a new car, a new life, a new outfit, to be someplace else, to try something new, to buy something new, a new medication, another massage, new furniture, a stiff drink; but nothing ever works, nothing will appease this restive appetite. We pace and feel suffocated. Maybe we need a new partner, a quick fling, a long vacation, ...*something, something.* It is a singular predicament of our Western culture that we can't ever seem to feel contented, relaxed, sated.

A positive feedback system is a system in which the data being studied responds to a disturbance by increasing the original data, in endless repetition. The end result of a positive feedback loop is thus amplifying. And since it is a repeating loop the disturbance itself will grow repeatedly larger. A simple example would be the effect of capitalizing the interest on an insurmountable loan. You are unable to pay the loan back, so it gains interest. The interest is "capitalized", meaning added to the original loan. Now the amount you owe is larger so your next interest payment is also larger. That is then added to the loan, and on and on. As you can see, the effect of a positive feedback loop is not necessarily "positive" in the sense of being desirable. A positive feedback loop can run out of control, and can result in the collapse of the system.

Eating poorly can be seen as the initiation of a positive feedback system if we acknowledge that we exist in an environment where the ability to acquire the appropriate nutrients is not available to many of us considering all the factors discussed in chapter one. In fact most, if not all of the last few generations may have actually been *born* into a nutritional version of this system, given that they may have been reared on formula, and raised in a time when the nutrients in even the best foods have declined markedly over the last hundred years.

Add to the mix that our air is polluted and our waters contain chemicals which never existed in nature, and you have an organism whose every cell is in a state of craving from its inception. The craving only grows. The nutritional deficits in our diet and the contamination of our environment compound this shortcoming more and more as we continue to subsist in the same conditions.

Is it any wonder that we, as a culture, overeat? We overindulge in countless other ways as well, trying to satisfy an unnamed hunger.

The entire spirit of America is considered by many to be one of lavish, driven, extravagance. We feel we need to compensate, console and comfort ourselves with food- because we work too hard, have no center, have no peace, don't get enough rest. Food is portrayed as a reward, becomes an ingrained solace for a life perceived of as not having enough rewards. We believe we are being short-changed constantly. And so we need to soothe ourselves with something cheap, easy, accessible, and slightly naughty. Something immediate. Something which fills a primal longing, an intangible unrelenting emptiness.

Who does it benefit to have us believe that we "deserve" more, that we should treat ourselves to an indulgence at every moment that is not a peak moment? Or that every moment should *be* a peak moment? It benefits the manufacturer of that in which we choose to indulge. It directly benefits someone else when we believe we haven't got enough, ever: Enough time, enough money, enough luxury, enough love.

How convenient for those chem-food cartels offering their products to fill that need. Do you think they know?

They know. You are being led.

There are corporations and industries duking it out for your dollar. We have not yet reached an era when there is a single power in control of all. But at this point in time it is already a frighteningly small handful of corporations who are vying to own our entire food supply,[20] from a seed or beaker to sani-wrapped, microwavable, cardboard facsimile of a meal. So do I think that it's all one big conspiracy? No, silly. But there are certainly many small conspiracies. This is a snowball which has become an avalanche as a result of a million little decisions picked up along the way.

Do I think that there are aloof scientists,[21] smarmy marketers, callous CEOs each of whom egotistically thinks of him or herself as a "P. T. Barnum" milking a gullible public? Yes. Do I think there are farmers, ranchers, growers, each of whom is aware that what they are doing is at least vaguely problematic, yet continues to do it "for the bottom line"? Yes. Do I think that there are inspectors, PR people, middle managers who know things aren't right, perhaps feel remorseful but rationalize their guilt in the name of self-interest and do it anyway? Yes. Do I think that there are cunning lawyers, cut-throat sales reps and scheming politicians who just don't care? Yes. Do I think all these people are getting together in one big room with an overarching evil blueprint to take over the world? Of course not. But the result is the same—we are destroying the gift of food which gives us life.

Dissimulation is the name of the game for industry lobbyists, for litigators, spokespeople and spin doctors (including the ever popular "Spin MDs" in newspapers and on television, supported by commercial sponsors). It's telling that there are, in fact, so many categories of employment in today's society whose sole purpose is obfuscation.

Corporations make every effort to skirt or circumvent or reinterpret the laws and the rules while their government lapdogs the USDA, the FDA and the EPA clear their path and fight off citizen whistleblowers and watchgroups. Even as I write this Tyson Foods, Inc. is in a lawsuit fighting a semantic argument over an antibiotic which it still feeds to its chickens while continuing to label and sell them as "Raised Without Antibiotics" for the past year.[22]

A corporation may be seen as a legal person in the eyes of the law, but, as famously stated by the English Baron Edward Thurlow, "Did you ever expect a corporation to have a conscience, when it has no soul to be damned, and no body to be kicked ?" Capitalism never looks back. Our system does not acknowledge it's past mistakes. When mistakes are made, rather than stop the process that created the mistakes, a "fix" is found and the relentless machine chugs on.

Our health is not the priority, no matter how many carefully constructed maudlin TV commercials they make —full of green valleys, pristine skies, laughing children and affluent cherry-cheeked elders enfolded by warm home-y flower gardens— in an effort to get us to believe that they are looking out for us or that they care about our children, our parents, our environment, our health or our quality of life.

In addition to the overwhelming number of people suffering from general malaise, according to government statistics each day in the US more than 200,000 people are directly sickened by something they ate, 900 are hospitalized, that's 76,000 people a year suffering from food poisoning, more than 5000 of them die. Those numbers are growing.

"A generation ago, the typical outbreak of food poisoning involved a small gathering: a church supper, a family picnic, a wedding reception. Contaminated food made a group of people in one local area get sick. Such traditional outbreaks still take place. But the nation's current system of food processing has created a whole new sort of outbreak, one that can potentially sicken millions of people." says Eric Shlosser.

In the past if you didn't like Guiseppi's zucchini, or were unsatisfied with his sanitation practices, you simply bought zucchini from Carlos or Bob, his neighbors. Or, of course, you grew your own. Today less than 2% of the population is responsible for growing our food. While this may seem terrific— the rest of us are free to do other things— what this means that we no longer can go to the next guy, there is no next guy. If Guiseppi found he was losing customers, he had to change his ways.

Today Guiseppi is a brand and a logo with a phalanx of lawyers, lobbyists, tacitly colluding political well-wishers and a multi-million dollar marketing team which includes the FDA and the USDA and can almost completely control what you have access to in the way of food and information about that food.

Frances Moore Lappe and daughter Anna discovered in research for their recent book *Hope's Edge* that economic markets "premised on highest return to existing wealth" controlled food supply and production and created a lack of food. "This is the first time in history that we are destroying the very basis of life itself, every piece of the atmosphere, soil, and water," says Lappe.

"The failure of agriculture," notes Vandana Shiva, author and

Indian food-sovereignty activist, (and a personal hero of mine), "is a success for the corporation."[23]

"Right now," states Howard Lyman, former cattle rancher turned vegetarian "we have governments that are doing the bidding of multinational corporations, and *they*, in fact, are the governments of the world."

In the words of the philosopher/ rapper/ poet who calls himself "New York Oil" we have become an "irresponsible culture" which makes a "business out of marketing evil."

We are overweight and overmedicated. Disease and the ravages of the physical decline of our bodies is evident everywhere in the Western world. We are being preyed upon yet seem to be quite oblivious and trusting as a whole, and especially when it comes to our food. Food is not *just* a health issue, though that should be of utmost importance to you, it is also a world security issue, an environmental issue, an issue of our survival. That our own health does not concern us until it's too late speaks volumes about the degradation of the human race as we have known it.

Traditional cultures are being destroyed, old ways of life being lost −most importantly, skills necessary for any culture anywhere in the world to be able to feed themselves are being lost (sometimes forcibly, but more often cunningly) and replaced by a dependence on the "authorities."

How did we get to a place where the majority of us have become cavalier about or resigned to so much destruction? What does it take to get us to notice? And why is it, when we do notice, we seem to expect someone else to straighten it out and clean it up?

CHAPTER 3

Surrendering the Keys to Dad

"I have seen the enemy, and he is us"
~ Pogo (Walt Kelly)

Beware those who would protect you for your own good, and who are profiting in the meanwhile, from their beneficence.

How is it, we asked in chapter two, that we have gotten to a point where we are so trusting of the quality of the food products we are eating that most of us have little clue about the processes involved in creating those food products? How can it be that our food has become such a boxed and packaged commodity that many of our children don't know that meat is from what had been a living animal? Or that vegetables came from the soil?

Most adults rarely pause to consider these facts when eating. We are insulated and removed from the labor and cycles of life which provide our very sustenance. Instead we are being virtually spoonfed like babies— someone else is preparing the food and all we have to do is open our mouths and pop it in (often with our hands, like babies) –and most of us seem to be ok with that.

"We're seeing the first fast-food generation that was brought up by a fast-food generation," said Elaine Ratner, publisher of *Now You're Cooking*,[1] a book meant to introduce neophytes to their kitchens. It's almost a cliché to hear a woman insist that she "just can't cook" and men have been trained to believe that cooking is "a woman's job" for at least the last century (except, ironically, when it comes to commanding a professional kitchen.)

In the year 2000 an average of one in five meals was eaten outside the home in America.[2] Although in today's current economic climate that figure has begun to shrink, people instead are turning to packaged prepared meals and/or grazing all day on snack foods.

Surrendering the Keys to Dad

Why do we almost universally seem to believe that we are incapable of cooking a dish or a meal from scratch, something that was commonplace a century ago? Most Americans would be completely lost attempting to grow their own food, no less butchering an animal. We do not feel confident in even planning our own diets. We need authority figures to tell us how to eat.

For that matter, most people do not know how to change their oil in their autos, flush their radiator or do basic maintenance on their vehicle, treat a simple cold or flu without the intervention of an authority (be it a medical professional or a pharmaceutical product), preserve their own surplus food, or care for themselves in even the most rudimentary way without a professional to do things for them.

Activities which used to be considered common knowledge for basic living are now considered survival skills, a hobby for fringe groups. If less than 2% of the population farms, this also means that 98% of us have lost the ability to sustain ourselves. More than 80.8% of the US population lives in an urban or suburban environment. Some people garden but many more do not. By choosing to relinquish the understanding and available space for growing your own food, you have given up much more than owning a gun, for instance. Talk about being able to defend yourself! You cannot defend your family if you are unable to even feed your family. And most people have lost the knowledge. Without a change in our habits we leave ourselves at the mercy of multinational corporations who have no interest in our national well-being or the continuance of our communities.

Today many Americans seem to express a certain pride in not expending any energy at all. It is seen as a measure of our success to hire others to do things for us like cleaning our houses, organizing our closets, walking our dog, making our phone calls, arranging our meetings. Someone else styles our hair, trims our nails, prepares our boxed convenience foods. We have become a nation who –astonishingly– *still* throws trash out the windows of our car rather than walk 20 feet to a receptacle. "Someone else will clean it up" is the belief. "Let someone else do it" is the motto of "Generation Me." We believe we're better than the kind of person who would have to do cleaning or pick up garbage. We are told we are more important, our time is more important, our needs, our comfort, our leisure is more important than that.

We purchase machines to do many jobs. We use sit-on lawnmowers for our 1500 sq. ft. lawns. We drive around the block to a neighbor's house. We make a point not to make a move or lift a finger. We don't want to get wet, cold, hot, ...up. Instead, we surround ourselves with "toys" and compete to see who has the most. We're living in a little playpen whose walls are getting smaller every day, but we're too busy, too mesmerized by the flashing lights, burbling sounds and bright colors of our trinkets and trifles to even notice.

Don't Touch That, Junior!
(Better let the "experts" handle it)

In this chapter I consider several watershed socio-political movements in US history which factor heavily into our current national sense of confusion and ineptitude regarding our own basic maintenance. It is my hope that in examining the trajectory of previous and parallel conditions in which we relinquished our autonomy, we can better understand how we reached our current state regarding our diet.

Prohibition

Prohibition in 1920s America seems to have been a big failure on the part of the those who were trying to outlaw alcohol. After much public outcry and more than a decade of speak-easys and rumrunners, the amendment banning alcohol was repealed in 1933 and things went back to the way they'd been. Or did they?

Not really. In past times many homesteads and estates brewed their own ales and beers and in some parts of the country immigrants from wine making countries made wines. Brewing is something that has been done in the home since pre-history as far back as almost 10,000 years. Actually, in all ancient cultures, from Mesopotamia to Peru, from Ethiopia to Egypt, women were the brew masters because brewing and bread making were considered part of the same craft. (By the way, it was considered a prestigious endeavor, not a chore, and men and women shared equally in the results.) Wine-making was often a community affair. The making of spirits is considerably newer, only several thousand years old, and has been accomplished by people from all walks of life.

Several of America's founding fathers brewed their own beer, including George Washington and Thomas Jefferson.[3] But as the US grew, just like in ancient cultures, drinking houses arose. In fact most of the concepts, tactics and allegiances of the American Revolution were formulated in taverns. As pubs proliferated in the early decades of the nineteenth century, the government, like governments throughout history, decided it wanted a piece of such a lucrative and commonplace activity. Alcohol taxes and tariffs were created. In the 1870s there were more than 4000 commercial breweries in the US, one hundred years later there were only 117, with less than 10 holding dominant market share.

In between was Prohibition. Laws prohibiting the manufacture of beer, wine or spirits imposed stiff fines on common people for an activity which had been commonplace for thousands of years. In hindsight Prohibition seems a ridiculous undertaking. Until one realizes two (among several) of the little-discussed, but profound changes it wrought. One- it swiftly and decisively consolidated the commercial manufacture of alcohol into a relatively few hands, the easier to tax and keep track of. Two- the home manufacture of beer (the easiest to do and most common alcoholic beverage) remained illegal for another 45 years. This further insured that nearly all alcohol consumption –something in which an ample percentage of households in almost all cultures historically engaged– would be taxed.

Importantly, it also created new generations of people who no longer had the skills to create their own alcohol. Now, creating alcohol isn't difficult and since the laws banning homebrew were changed in 1978 (by most states, it is still illegal in Alabama) to allow small batches to be made, there are a small but growing number of hobbyists experimenting in this arena. Before this change there was a vague but widespread belief among common people that "you'd go blind" or worse, if attempting to make your own alcohol. In fact there are websites today with heated discussion of the dangers of home distilling even among those hobbyists who make wine or beer.[4]

What really happened during that drought of information and hands-on knowledge is that people began to believe that they couldn't do it themselves. The newly burgeoning mass media of the 1920s, with the advent of radio, had played a huge roll in convincing people that their own ineptitude in the making of alcohol was the cause of countless cases of blindness, illness and death with stories of bathtub gin and other illicit booze destroying lives. This was natural since the substance was illegal and popular media coverage then, like now, is prone to elaborate a specific point of view, and not one that goes against the government on legal issues if they want to stay in business. Horror stories abounded. Yet most of the illness and injury was actually caused by unscrupulous vendors who adulterated their product for profit.[5] When Prohibition was over the fears remained. Alcohol became readily available in pubs again, it was illegal to make at home and so it had become something that most people no longer did for themselves. Many had begun to believe that it was difficult to do or required things they didn't have. Almost all, consciously or not, decided that it was best left to professionals.

The AMA

Even long before the Prohibition years, changes were taking place within this new society that were more subtle and less noticeable to the average homesteader or townsperson. In the earliest part of the nineteenth century communities were far more widely dispersed than they are now. The necessity of self-sufficiency in every important aspect of life was the norm, as well as a strong interdependency on one's neighbors. The need for community was paramount.

There were people in nineteenth century America who might never have come in contact with a medical doctor. Communities relied on their elder women for most medical care, doctors were often out of reach in urban areas or only available to the wealthy. Says Jane Allured in a document on the history of rural America: "In most nineteenth century communities, female healers performed almost all of the tasks that professionally trained doctors, nurses, and pharmacists later assumed."[6]

She quotes a resident of resident of Taney County, Missouri about the situation as recently as the early 20 century:

> "The nearest doctor was 20 miles away and there was no way to travel only horseback and no money to pay with if he did come. . . . Mother watched over us carefully. There wasn't money to buy medicine."

This person goes on to describe the treatments and preparations her mother used to keep the family well. Ms. Allured through her research, tells us, "domestic medicine was an almost exclusively feminine art, passed down from mother to daughter." Women relied on each other for advice and experience and their families relied on them. The most experienced in any given region was apt to become the local midwife. Midwifery was the mainstay of normal childbirth for so many centuries that it is even mentioned in the Bible.

Although midwives and the wisdom of women's experience was valued within the community, the prestige of an educated male from the big city (men being seen as having higher status in general) attracted those who could afford to call for a doctor.

By the early 1800s, when one did have the means to visit a professional there were two main schools of medical treatment, what we now call "conventional" or orthodox medicine and Homeopathy. Orthodox, or allopathic medicine had been around for some time and was the providence of wealthy males who had acquired a university degree of the time.

According to the FDA's website:

> "In the late 1700s, the most popular therapy for most ailments was bloodletting. Some doctors had so much faith in bleeding that they were willing to remove up to four-fifths of the patient's blood.

Other therapies of choice included blistering--placing caustic or hot substances on the skin to draw out infections--and administering dangerous chemicals to induce vomiting or purge the bowels.

Massive doses of a mercury-containing drug called calomel cleansed the bowels, but at the same time caused teeth to loosen, hair to fall out, and other symptoms of acute mercury poisoning. Homeopathy is a medical theory and practice that developed in the late 1700/early 1800s in reaction to the bloodletting, blistering, purging, and other harsh procedures of conventional medicine as it was practiced more than 200 years ago." [7]

Paul Starr, in *The Social Transformation of American Medicine*, notes: "There is general agreement among medical historians today that orthodox medicine of the 1700s and 1800s in particular frequently caused more harm than good." [8]

Homeopathy gained rapid popularity because of its gentler approach and because of homeopathic doctor's insistence on "simples"— the use of only one element at time for a given condition as opposed to the concoctions of apothecaries (evolved from alchemists) who provided orthodox doctors with their treatments. The middle and lower classes (as well as many in the upper classes) found these simples at least equally effective, less destructive to the body and significantly cheaper to acquire. Homeopathic doctors, often from the same universities as orthodox doctors, began to be widely and loudly disparaged by members of the orthodoxy, especially as they gained favor throughout the population, claiming notable advocates such as Thomas Jefferson, Mark Twain, Harriet Beecher Stowe, Daniel Webster, William James, Henry Wadsworth Longfellow, Nathanial Hawthorne, Horace Greeley, and Louisa May Alcott.

So when the homeopathic upstarts (according to allopathic doctors) formed the American Institute of Homeopathy in 1844 it was seen as a looming threat to conventional medicine. Likewise, says the *Wellness Directory of Minnesota*, "As the population of doctors grew, so did their desire to put midwives out of business and take over their practices." [9]

Surrendering the Keys to Dad

In rapid response, by 1847, orthodox practitioners formed the American Medical Association (AMA). Members of the AMA, drawn from the upper classes, were alarmed at all the other schools of medicine —but especially homeopathy which had the fastest growing following and midwifery which was universal— who were competing for the hearts and minds and pocketbooks of those who could afford a genuine city doctor. Their primary concern was that they were suffering economically as a result. In *Healing the Health-Care System*, Lawrence D. Wilson, MD, states: "Perhaps the most important reason that conventional physicians disliked homeopathy and homeopaths was well expressed at an AMA meeting by one of the more respected orthodox physicians who said, 'We must admit that we never fought the homeopath on matters of principles; we fought him because he came into the community and got the business.'" [10]

The AMA was quickly supported by the Apothecaries Union who shared in their resentment of homeopathic doctors for the "stealing" their income, through the homeopaths' avoidance of caustics and purgatives and complex apothecary concoctions.

The AMA also enjoyed the backing of their longstanding patrons, those of status and means within the urban areas where medical doctors were usually found. This enabled them to pressure their peers, the lawyers and politicians, to enact laws declaring all other forms of healing besides their own as unlawful. In their push for control even obstetrics and gynecology began to be practiced by "regular" doctors as they called themselves, in spite of great public outcry at the perceived indecency as well as the absurdity of men performing these functions. "We cannot deny that women possess superior capacities for the science of medicine," wrote Samuel Thomson, a Health Movement leader, in 1834. [11]

Although respect was accorded the position of sage-femme, or healing woman, within each household inasmuch as she was called upon and responsible for the health of its members, the role was not the equivalent of a doctor or even a midwife as we know them today. For one thing it was not a position of prestige. A woman simply kept her family well in the same fashion in which her husband kept his livestock cared for; it was what you did. A woman outside the home considered particularly knowledgeable might be called upon for cases out of the ordinary, where her longer years of experience might prove useful. Her grateful beneficiaries might provide a meal or a chicken.

The average female head of household used an understanding of local plants, primarily, which had been passed down from her mother or aunt or neighbor, in addition to as varied and healthful a diet as could be gotten in her circumstances.

Then, as now, inability to access a decent diet was usually a result of politics, rarely paucity. Though often certain species of meats or exotic spices or plants were kept by the wealthy for themselves, what we call "wild" plants were commonly eaten as potherbs and, except in cases of dire oppression or calamitous weather, the diet of past centuries was much more varied then we often imagine it. (It was also usually far more varied than our own.)

And so the housewife had many remedies: broths, syrups, tinctures, poultices, salves, compresses, teas, and herbs at her disposal in addition to whole grains, fresh meats and locally grown vegetables with which to keep her household well. Even treats in most cultures were as often savory as sweet. The distinction our culture makes between food as merely filling one's belly and food for health was almost nonexistent. The act of preparing a meal engaged the entire family and was a shared blessing of life and health.

The AMA fought ruthlessly to seize control of all forms of what it deemed "medical practice" and disparage all competitors, despite not having a noticeable success rate of patient recoveries themselves. Relentlessly, viciously attacking their perceived adversaries' practices as "immoral", "quackery", and "fraudulent," they forced homeopaths and women from universities, denied them a license to practice medicine, forbade them from any activity which could be construed as practicing medicine. Nonetheless, mothers and other women within communities, especially rural communities, black communities, and immigrant communities, continued to be viewed as valuable sources of healing and knowledge. Homeopaths, herbalists, midwives and other healers continued to be embraced by the mainstream –until medicine found collusion with the petrochemical industry.

> "It was discovered in the late 19th century that the by-products of petroleum refinement could be used to manufacture synthetic chemicals and drugs. Production of pharmaceuticals grew with the development of the petrochemical industry. *'If doctors could be persuaded to reorient medicine towards the norm of pharmacotherapy (cure by drugs),'* points out Professor of Law and Medicine Ian Kennedy, *'then clearly here were riches indeed.'* Institutions like the Rockefeller Foundation which stemmed from Standard Oil (Exxon), donated massive sums of money to guide medical education around the turn of the century. Pharmacology became integral to the curriculum, medicine an indispensable tool of the doctor."[12]

As the nation entered the 20th century, members of the AMA really turned up the pressure, acquiring organized philanthropy in the form of foundations, like the Rockefeller Foundation, created by their advocates. These foundations then crafted reports for the public exclaiming the unassailable superiority of allopathic medicine, in tactics very much like those in use today.

Slightly more than a decade after WWI there began an exponential increase in the manufacture of synthetic chemical medical treatments, as an outgrowth of the chemical industries built during the war. Coupled with the assiduous self promotion of the AMA, with laws medical professionals had managed to have enacted, and the concurrent discovery of antibiotics, the imminent extinction of anything other than orthodox medicine was nearly accomplished.

The public was finally strong-armed into believing that the governance of their health should be turned over to the hands of someone within the single remaining legal medical channel, a medical doctor, and that it was dangerous and foolhardy to do otherwise. Through media promotion, the image of medical science was intimately entwined with the exhilarating belief, in that period, in "better living through chemistry" and the noble, paternal doctor. Surely he knew more than we ever would. Care of our own health was something with which the average person no longer felt capable.

The Kitchen

Although we often think of different countries or regions as having a stable and [uniform] cultural body of foods, the fact is that every culture's food palette has continually evolved throughout history. What is noteworthy in modern Western culture is the speed at which those changes happen.

In the past, change happened at a glacial pace- one century might introduce cinnamon but it might take a generation or longer before the spice was widely used within that culture. The next century would see the introduction of chocolate or artichokes and then these novelties would slowly insinuate themselves into the menu over the course of decades.

All of that changed in 20th century America. By the 1950s, explosive population growth, the noteworthy success of various immigrant communities, the flourishing of suburban neighborhoods in the United States, the introduction and growth of mass media, the automobile with its enticing invitation to new horizons, fast food joints which dotted the landscape, the rapidly expanding chemical and pharmaceutical industries as an outgrowth of the wars, and the incipient economic boom as well as the baby boom were simultaneously a result of and indicative of American's sudden sense of the accessibility of anything. Synthetic materials beckoned in every realm – new fabrics, plastic dishware, cheap appliances, toys, synthetic drugs, synthetic fertilizers; everywhere was growth and the expectation of growth.

The national sense was that of a people on the move. It was the era of the Jet Set, the Space Race. Factories churning, wheels rolling, exponential increases in agricultural production, everything seemed limitless, yet within our grasp. If we didn't have it we could make it in a lab. There was a collective breath of freedom, a lifting of the ties to the cold dark uncertain decades past with their World Wars and Depression, hardships, rationing, and crowded multi-generational households.

Suddenly entire neighborhoods were often made up of young couples away from home for the first time, away from the guidance and oversight, stability and cynicism of their elders. The old world ways of their parents were shed much the way traditional garments and habits had been. This was a new America, young, bright, bustling, and exuding (if not quite always feeling) confidence.

Into this giddy heady time, exciting innovations in cooking became increasingly available to the average shopper. Starry-eyed suburbanites were perfect fodder for the savvy advertising agencies whose tactics were coming of age, advocating all manner of quick-fix products nationally via the exciting and suddenly ubiquitous medium of television. Frozen foods, TV dinners, instant coffee, Kool-aid, cake mixes, Tang; food products promoted the fast paced self image embraced by people who saw themselves as busy forging the future from new fabric.

And if these sometimes unfamiliar food products presented challenges to the young cooks who'd never encountered them before, the advertising agencies filled the void— they became the trusted guides, the ersatz elder sibling/ mom/ wizened aunt. They were glitzy barkers for the new American panorama: a world of our own making.

> "Even as Americans became more and more widely dispersed geographically, they became more and more a single nation, all making the same recipes found on the backs of boxes. Betty Crocker represented a new kind of authority, acting *in loco parentis.*"
>
> –Thomas Hine, *Populuxe* [13]

Yes, Betty Crocker and all the other brands of the day, as well as magazines and television began to lend a solicitous hand in the kitchen. And they were indispensable. Grandmother certainly wasn't going to teach you how to make a green bean casserole with cream of mushroom soup and a can of French's fried onion topping or a lime gelatin ring with fried spam and canned pineapple, filled with cottage cheese. Only a modern housewife reading the latest magazines had access to recipes like these.

In an article for the Illinois Times about 1950's fare, Julianne Glatz states: "The advertising made homemakers feel as if they had to use packaged convenience foods if they wanted to keep up with the times. Newspaper columns, 'women's' magazines, and daily radio programs hosted by such luminaries as 'Harriet Hepplewhite, the Happy Housewife' assured their audience that cooking from scratch was hopelessly outdated."

This fabricated anxiety about being behind the times has gone from "out-of-season" to not "up-to-the-minute." The pace has quickened. It plies on our fear of rejection. We are emphatically told that there is a "norm" for ways of doing and being, and warned with foreboding that we might be committing an embarrassing faux pas without even being aware of it.

The implication is that we might find ourselves shunned or outcast. We're imbued with the idea that there is only one way to cook or to eat, and we can't know what it is without their help. Like the '50s housewife who feared being labeled hopelessly outdated and struggled to maintain a modern kitchen, we are assured that we won't fit in if we don't seek out and comply with the latest prescribed meals and methods.

A favorite example of this is a contemporary Lean Cuisine television commercial where several women describe their horrible dinner the night before, things like three donuts and a diet soda, a grapefruit and a 20 oz. bag of potato chips and the like, as a way of bonding.

One woman describes in great detail what seems to be a lavish meal with fresh vegetables and a meat and pasta entrée. Her friends stop bonding, even stop in their tracks — the music stops— and they look at her with betrayal and suspicion in their expressions, until she reveals that it is a frozen prepared meal from a box. Only then is she accepted back into the fold. In this case we are encouraged to believe that preparation of a balanced meal with a real entrée and vegetables will be viewed with wariness and reproach. It is seen as one-upmanship, a threat to one's peer group. Today's woman doesn't have time for that. *Who do you think you are?*

"During the postwar era, time became an obsession of the food industry and eventually of American homemakers as a manufactured sense of panic began to pervade even day-to-day cooking. Advertisements and stories plowed across the media reminding readers again and again how busy they were, how frantic their days, how desperately they needed products and recipes for quick meals," says Laura Shapiro, in her book "*Something From the Oven.*"

Does that "manufactured sense of panic" sound familiar? You know the tune: your life is harried, hurried, hectic, frantic: boom boom boom —it's still being played to us. But advertisers weren't about to settle for a one note song.

The shocking realization of American's poor heart health in the sixties, scientist's newly established link between high blood cholesterol levels and heart disease and the entrenched competition of growing food industry giants suddenly introduced a new concern into our food choices—controversy over health benefits. Packaged convenience had become established. Fast food was well ensconced in our national self image. The question was no longer whether to consume these food products, only which ones.

Over the ensuing decades facets of the market began jostling to create food products which would be perceived by the public as being healthier choices, often for reasons which seemed to change daily. Enemies lists were drawn and fought bitterly over. Salt was suddenly one day seen as Satan's condiment. Margarine was ballyhooed over butter. Low fat, no fat/ low-salt, no salt became all the rage. Diets proliferated in which natural fats were replaced with margarines, salt erased from some lifestyles entirely (sometimes to the dieter's detriment).

Then we were informed that carbohydrates, something most

people only knew from seventh grade science class, had become the new opponent. Breads and pasta, potatoes, oatmeal, rice were all banished from the modern menu of the time. Later, for a while, MSG was on everybody's lips. Then nitrates and cyclamates. America's insatiable sweet tooth was mollified with a flurry of synthetic sweeteners- each of them became a controversy.

Long gone were the days when food had ethnic or regional significance (though that has been brought back in caricature by marketers of our own era). No longer were meals simply about balance or even creativity, now there was daily controversy about each ingredient. Medical professionals, nutrition experts, diet gurus— all were aligned in various camps, expounding and extrapolating.

The media changed sides routinely, with bright-eyed sincerity at each turn. New words and phrases popped up faster than tornados in Kansas: low-fat, lean, lite, saturated fats, nitrites, nitrates, cyclamates, cholesterols, triglycerides, trans-fats, probiotics, body mass, olestra, antioxidants, aspartame, sucralose, tagatose, BHA; and on and on.

Packages became plastered over with meaningless claptrap like "gluten-free margarine," "light oil," "zero trans fat soda," to make you believe that the product inside is somehow healthful, while asserting nothing.

People often sincerely tried to make healthy choices, based on the knowledge of the moment, only to find out with the next medical revelation that they'd been all wrong. We were told over and over to read ingredient labels, yet it was repeatedly revealed that the labels had been made deliberately misleading or research found them to be full of chemical nomenclature that meant nothing to the average consumer.

In the last few decades, it has begun to seem that only someone with an advanced degree: a doctor or a chemist or a nutritionist is capable of knowing the right ingredients, in the proper amounts to keep us healthy. Television and magazines employ doctors and nutritionists as a regular feature to explain the daily-changing intricacies of diet. Who else could know what has the correct balance of ..."good" things, and what is free of the fickle list of "bad" things? If we can no longer trust our senses, where do we turn? The average consumer, in order to know which things are safe and what is no longer ok to eat, is now expected to rely on the authorities to inform us.

These same authorities, in various guises, are currently working to restrict our access to nature's herbs, unprocessed milk, raw almonds and more, while lowering the bar on organic standards at the insistence of big corporations and acknowledging that it is impossible to prevent nationwide outbreaks of the now-familiar bugs E. coli and salmonella and the like, in our unwieldy industrial food system.

These same authorities suggest that we put our eight-year-olds on statin drugs as their little bodies begin to spiral out of control. Many regular, ordinary people have decided that it's time to take back the reins of our own lives.

CHAPTER 4

The Endless Child

"People are like stained-glass windows.
They sparkle and shine when the sun is out, but
when the darkness sets in their true beauty is
revealed only if there is a light from within."
~ Elizabeth Kubler-Ross

In the past people depended on each other, it was all they had. While a "barn-raising" has become something of a cliché, in fact barns as well as every other building were all built by gatherings of neighbors. Planting, harvesting, birthing, healing, the pressing of oil, the making of wine, in all affairs we were intricately tied to our family members and our local network, our community. And all activities were tied to the seasons: hogs butchered (a group activity) at a certain time of the year, beef or rabbit, venison, chicken, squirrel eaten at other times; greens picked during some months, fruit picked during others.

Children were given jobs relative to their abilities and were seen as –and felt themselves to be– valued, integral members of the clan and village. Even non-farm village shops and crafts work incorporated all ages of people, these enterprises were often an extension of the home. Life wasn't all brutal hardship. There was time for oral histories, tales and stories, music making, singing, dance, intimacy and connection. Yes, there was disease, but there is still disease. There was grief and heartbreak, but there is still grief and heartbreak.

We are reminded constantly of the gains we have made in the 20th and 21st centuries, but often we overlook the price we've had to pay. The era of industrialization began to not only isolate us in terms of men and women leaving home to work in factories, but exacerbated gender segregation as well as removing children from daily active participation in the maintenance of the family's well-being.

The automobile served to further detach us from nature: it has cut us off from the lives of the animals that we used to depend upon. By not interacting with other species, witnessing their relationships with each other, their cycles of life and death, we have lost immeasurable insight into our own lives. By not tangibly depending on other species we have ended up trivializing their lives and have further emotionally extracted ourselves from our genuine place in the fabric of life. According to Edith Hood, a spokesperson for the Navaho nation, the Navajo have a concept called "hozho."

> "Hozho is how we live our lives. It means balance, beauty and harmony between we, the five-fingered people, and nature. When this balance is disturbed, our way of life, our health and our wellbeing all suffer."[1]

We are suffering. The unprecedented mobility offered by the automobile intensified the dissolution of the extended family and did away with the foundations of stable communities. It spurred an internal American diaspora whose turbulence has only increased as people now relocate not once, but many times in the course of their lives.

We are no longer tied to seasons. Living in climate controlled environments with synthetic light, we have lost the mystery of the night. We are sold fabricated foodstuffs and have no idea what they're made from. Our refrigerators and freezers and that ubiquitous "shelf life" have banished the rhythm of the real urgency of meals −rapid decay− which demanded that the food we ate was always at its freshest, the better to provide the nutrients we need.

The age of technology has estranged us even further from each other, from nature, from ourselves. At what point does the ceaseless succession of flashing images from our television and computer screens become hypnotic? We are bombarded with imagery and noises which keep us constantly distracted, yet we don't make the connection to a stupendous spectrum of disorders related to inattention, inability to focus and just general twitchiness. [*Maybe we can't because we're always distracted...*] We are experiencing a species overload.

We are so removed from the cycle of life that we are lost. Most disturbing is the fact that we cannot even recognize this loss, we don't know what is missing because modern generations have never had it. We are so disoriented as a culture that we have become a nation of pill-poppers hoping to quell the anxiety born of this state of being untethered from our connection to the Earth: that which grounds us. Still, we are encouraged by advertisers to placate ourselves with playthings while being inundated with soothing assurances that we are safe, that it's all ok. That we are being protected. That science, the authorities, have the answers.

Marketing —all marketing— is based on fear. Fear of rejection, of being uncool, or unattractive, fear of not being included, fear of being alone, fear of not "making it"- not being seen as successful or valuable- of not having achieved the right degree or status, fear of illness, fear of making mistakes in caring for our children, fear of age, fear of losing all we have to catastrophe or through misstep.

Marketing plays expertly to those very human self-doubts. By making the focus of our lives entirely about ourselves —removed from symbiosis with nature, with spirituality, with the larger external issues which held past generations— we have developed blinders to our larger connection with all of life.

All religions and many culture's allegorical folklore warn of the dangers of hubris. Vanity and excess pride used to be frowned upon within the populace in the same way that gluttony was once frowned upon. Only 200 years ago very few ordinary people even had mirrors hanging in their homes. Today we in the West appear to be a society of obsessed narcissists, where practically every phone and wristwatch comes with a camera for our self portraits.

In directing the whole of our attention to a single storm we fail to notice the relative stability of the coming and going of seasons. In directing the whole of our attention to a single skin blemish, we fail to notice even the storm. Instead of a vast miracle of a million stars dwarfing our egos and twinkling a little perspective on our tiny place in the world, we now have bright lights, billboards and glass towers reflecting only ourselves back at us, inflating us with precarious conceit. We can't see the forest for... ourselves.

By creating an atmosphere of relentless self absorption, we

have become a people who constantly chase an unattainable perfection. Perfect fodder for those trying to sell it to us. We are prodded to spend billions on appearance, be it younger skin, baldness remedies, breast implants, Viagra, faster cars, fashions, gadgets or gizmos. We have been fixated on our fear of our own imperfections, and endlessly urged to assuage our desires.

I am reminded of a another TV commercial which depicts a mother in the kitchen devouring her favorite sweetened breakfast cereal by the handful right out of the box while her husband and children pound desperately on the barricaded door begging her to share. There are countless spin-offs of the same theme: get it for *you*, save it in a hiding place just for *you*. The message that "It is all about you" has become a mantra for advertisers. We are encouraged to indulge our basest selves— our child-selves, even at the expense of our own children. We have become infantilized; we are the sun, the center of the universe. We are pressured and guided to live the life of The Endless Child.

Not surprisingly, in an analogous development, our foodstuff has been manufactured with an increasing emphasis on sweetness and blandness over the last several decades. Unlike adults of previous centuries, in all cultures, who preferred to experiment with piquant, tart, peppery, pungent, bitter, sour and countless other subtle distinctions of flavor, today's Western adults like our food sweet or salty and often otherwise flavorless.

It is not news that we are a "gimme, gimme, gimme" culture, but it has become more than simple selfishness. We are encouraged to think of ourselves as separate from and in competition with our neighbors and associates, even family members. Car commercials openly gloat about gleefully leaving the other guy in the dust. An entire genre of television show consists of people being harangued and humiliated.

This is not a message about winning a good fight or triumphing over tragedy or evil. It's about hoarding and greed, contempt for others. Exemplified by the ignoble behavior of John McEnroe in tennis, sports figures indulge public temper tantrums, throwing rackets, helmets, bicycles, bats and often punches. Celebrities rage at the paparazzi on whom they depend. Shoppers brawl over coveted baubles. We're shown the footage over and over again. A type of paranoia is created, we are egged on to believe that every encounter is a potential threat to one's ego, or one's all important immediate gratification. Snatching a "toy" from another "contestant" is fair game: you win, they lose.

In fact, to view ourselves through the mirror of the media, it appears that we've become a culture which exalts in what Christianity has called "The Seven Deadly Sins":

Pride is excessive belief in one's own abilities. It has been called the sin from which all others arise. Pride is also known as Vanity.

Envy is the desire for others' traits, status, abilities, or situation.

Gluttony is an inordinate desire to consume more than that which one requires.

Lust is an inordinate craving for the pleasures of the body.

Anger is manifested in the individual who spurns love and opts instead for fury. It is also known as Wrath.

Greed is the desire for material wealth or gain, ignoring the realm of the spiritual. It is also called Avarice or Covetousness.

Sloth is the avoidance of physical or spiritual work.[2]

It reads like a Wall Street/ business school personal ethics manifesto.

In every war the news media has singled out those whom we called the enemy and, with varying degrees of subtle or overt propaganda, demonized them, highlighted their differences from us, made them seem "other," aberrant, inferior. The difference is that now this tactic is being used to isolate us from our neighbor, our family, the community. This is a "divide and conquer" maneuver.

We have been urged to see ourselves as incapable of concentration while being blasted from every direction by a pulsing drumbeat of fleeting and contradictory advertisement and advice. (Who *could* concentrate in that environment?) Our bodies are rebelling from years of neglect and inadequate nutrients so that we spend much of our time feeling ill, dazed. We have been sold on instant gratification and repeatedly told that we are incapable of restraint until we have come to believe it. "We can't stop ourselves, we can't help it. It is not our fault;" so goes the zeitgeist of the last several decades. And always we are admonished that we are slipping behind, that someone else is going to get our piece of the pie.

Suburban and urban living isolates us from one another in the way that Western culture practices it. Our houses and apartments are discrete kingdoms, windows closed in the comfort of air conditioning, our doors locked. Often we don't know our neighbors. Everyone is a stranger. It is not uncommon that we enter and leave our residences in our automobiles from behind closed garage doors. Our communities are additionally segregated by age group; young people grow up and move out, older people are either left behind or move intentionally into age-segregated "senior" communities. Knowledge is no longer passed down, it is passed across the Internet. The generations don't share a history. Children often don't know their grandparents in any real sense. The ties that bind are typically consumer products: Hallmark cards, holiday gifts.

If we feel truly alone we are more vulnerable to exploitation. And exploitation is marketing's middle name.

The concept of the teenager is a prime example of a whole-y invented demographic, a manufactured emotional insecurity at an age when people used to be welcomed into the tribe. The idea of the teenager did not exist 100 years ago. In many non-Western cultures, it still does not exist today. Yet in the West, combined with the even newer demographic "Tweens" it is one of the largest target markets for fashion, shoes, electronics, junk food, music, and other frivolities of disposable income.

We have come to see teens, and now tweens, as discrete from other age groups and the attendant cliché of teen rebellion as predetermined, even by teens themselves who, of course, are bombarded with this same message. The teen, we are told, wants different clothes, different music, different food, and inhabits a different world, continually necessitating new product lines and new twists on old products which require new purchases.

It is significant that there is growing violence and angst among young people who are ready to be seen as worthwhile participants in our adult society, yet are told they must wait years for entrance and acceptance. They are instead exhorted to purchase a sense of belonging by buying into a fabricated peergroup purgatory of retail in which they can never have enough, or be enough. They are, in this way, deftly prepared for the adulthood of The Endless Child. And yet it is often in adolescence that people most keenly feel the shallow superficiality of the model that is being introduced to them. I suspect that is why the advertisers have begun to target younger and younger prey.

"I don't want to eat broccoli so I just won't, so there." This is a paraphrase of a famous statement made by a president of the US, George Bush the *first*, in a classic example of petulant "Endless Child" speak. "I got this body eating chocolate every day," a current diet spokeswoman insists. "I want ice cream everyday. I want pizza everyday. Its too hard to cook. I don't like it, I don't want to!" These are the messages rained upon us by advertisers and repeated by everyone in society right up through recent Presidents. They have been drummed into our subconscious. We throw up our arms in (childish) frustration at the conflicting messages and decide we're just gonna eat whatever we want. So there.

In this frenetic, egotistical, avaricious environment, we become easy prey for the next distraction, the next shiny object that is dangled in front of us. We naturally feel an urgency in the excitement and the hype, the shouts of the ringmaster, it is human instinct. We are then patted on the head and consoled about our so-called weaknesses with the message that it is happening to everybody and these are the products to buy, the drugs to take. All the while we are seduced by advertisement to continue the unhealthy diet, take more medications and, like children, to go ahead and eat that ice cream if we want it—
"you deserve it, we wouldn't tell you anything that would hurt you, we

care." Just don't consider getting off the Merry-Go-Round or you will risk becoming a social outcast. "Just trust us," is the message we keep getting.

Science has become our shaman. We follow blindly. White lab coats have become the equivalent of the village witch doctor's magical chicken-claw amulet. A white lab coat gives the wearer special powers. We attach more significance to his or her pronouncements when the person wears one. Most people don't know what all the big chemical words in our ingredient lists are, and more importantly they don't —couldn't be expected to— understand what meaning they have for our health. Many of the words on our food packages are literally hocus pocus. As with the shamans of old, we are trained to respond to the paraphernalia of the position- in this case the microscope, the stethoscope, the lab coat, an image of the pristine white and chrome room where mysteries outside the realm of our understanding take place. We must learn to recognize and see through this pageantry.

Another typical marketing tactic is exemplified by a phrase that Dannon has used on their yogurt products. It says "No Artificial Anything. ™ " That little "TM" means that the phrase is a trademark, not that it has any bearing whatsoever on the content of the container. (And in fact, that particular product contained artificial ingredients. Did you even notice the "TM"? No? That's just what they were counting on.) Other label words are newly minted marketing bon *mots* dreamt up by giddy junior execs in glass offices with the intent of sounding healthful and scientific but which are actually meaningless. If the words sound scientific, studies have shown that we will follow. When you read about the supposed health claims of decoy foods like Captain Kootie's Sugar Tooties or whatever the latest garbage is, think of a roomful of overpaid smirking 20-year olds sitting in some fancy office chortling as they come up with concepts that they are convinced will fool or befuddle you enough to purchase or pay more for their products.

In most older cultures much was made of an afterlife and correspondingly, one's behavior in this life. In this way people's proclivity towards selfishness, gluttony and other anti-social behavior was kept at bay, those inclinations were overtly frowned upon by those in power (and thus nearly everyone else down through society) because individuals needed to work together. Our culture, on the contrary, appears to want to foster these behaviors. "Now" is all that seems to count in our culture. Again—advertising. "Who has time to think of tomorrow?" we're told. In the social structure that we have in place, someone is benefiting from having us clash and jostle.

We have been conditioned to believe it's all about us and urged to see everyone else as beating us to the punch. That we will lose if we don't "punch" first—without thinking. (You'll miss the moment, you'll backslide, lose momentum, or fall short if you stop to reflect.) We have been proselytized into this mindset by the most powerful single evangelical group in the world—corporate advertisers.

It is natural to think of one's self and one's safety. And it is human instinct to measure one's self against the crowd, a way that we keep social norms. But it is a perversion of these innate propensities that we turn on each other in a confused inability to satisfy either our comfort level or our social standing. It is extremely unnatural for any animal and especially a human animal to soil it's bed or poison it's own food, yet we have been doing both.

Why? Because we have been giving up the mastery of our lives to someone else, perhaps without really being aware of it. Slowly, over time, piece by piece, for our own good, our own safety, for many of the theoretically right reasons, for some of the selfishly wrong ones, and sometimes unwittingly; we have been persuaded, cajoled and coerced to hand over control to so-called "authorities" that they may relieve us of the consequences of responsibility, the burdens of adulthood.

Beneath a facade of kindly paternalism, there has been a gradual, tyrannical sapping of our trust in ourselves. We are told that this is what *we* want. I'm not buying that. It's time to send them the message that you are not a child.

We are being portrayed as weak-willed impulse buyers, incapable of restraint. I'm not buying that.

86

The Endless Child

We are being portrayed as insatiably selfish, rapacious people. As people who don't have time to care about the bigger issues. We are portrayed as people who are incapable of discerning what is healthy for ourselves and our families.

We are being portrayed as being helplessly, irrevocably, addicted to junk foods. I'm not buying that.

We are being portrayed as people who can be tricked into believing that spreading toxic waste on our soil is a form of recycling, that we are a society who can't make the connection between the destruction of our habitat and the degradation of our species, that we are so self-engrossed that we will destroy our own children's future for our own immediate gratification and for the sake of convenience.

This is not the image of people that I see in America. I see a multifaceted movement that has already begun on many different fronts. I see people who care about the future, the planet, their children and our sustenance. "I'm not buying that." This is already the de-facto motto of this movement.

We are depicted in commercials as being a people who will accept low quality food-like products just because we are too lazy to take responsibility for our own lives. Tell the advertisers: "I'm not buying that."

When you go into the grocery store and are lured by a colorful box of powdered, reconstituted, enriched, dolled-up, dressed-up, worthless, nutrition-less crap, (with a long shelf life!) pause, take a breath, and say to yourself: "I'm not buying that."

When you walk past a fast food joint with its vents intentionally installed to waft its familiar smells over you at a mall or city street because they are so sure that you will react like an unrestrained infant and immediately want to satisfy that baby voice inside which says "Mmmmm, Eat!" though you're not even hungry, say to that voice, "I'm not buying that."

If you pass a junk food restaurant in your car and its flashing lights and super-duper discounts try to convince you that you are saving money or time by eating their unhealthy, greasy, over-salted cardboard products, think to yourself: "I'm not buying that." (*You* know the costs are much higher in the long term.)

When they offer you coupons, swear that it really is good for you, that scientists will back them up, or that everyone else is doing it, remain firm in your conviction: "I'm not buying that."

When they offer you pills, gels, liquids and prescriptions in order to hide from yourself the consequences of their unhealthy fare, say "No, I'm not buying that."

When they bring on the celebrities that they've been able to buy who try to convince you that it's uncool or misguided or just not fun, that nobody your age is really all that concerned about food because it's more popular to be irreverent, think to yourself, "I'm not buying that."

When they tell you your kids will be spurned, your husband mocked by his co-workers, that your friends will shun you, that you are doing your family a disservice by not shopping in "conventional" markets and buying processed decoy food products, say to yourself: "I'm not buying that."

When they tell you about studies which show that conventional food-products are safer, more consistent, subject to far more scrutiny, regulation and testing, know in your gut that they are trying to sell you a bill of goods and think: "I'm not buying that."

When news media (owned, of course, by its sponsors) begins to suggest that turning away from conventional foods is bad for the economy, will bring down the country, is the reason prices are so high; know that those sponsors want you to sacrifice yourself on the alter of *their* financial gain, and tell them: "I'm not buying that."

When they really turn up the heat— when they have medical professionals coming on air in white coats and somber expressions to warn you that you will become ill, your spouse will become angry, your children will hate you, ... tell them to go to hell.

That's right. What if we all decided to become well? To stand up to the onslaught of advertisement? What would happen to the billions and trillions spent on the medications that we stuff down to enable us to eat the things that are actually making us suffer? What if we could throw away the drugs for depression, anxiety and the inability to focus or concentrate? What if we all suddenly had a moment of perfect clarity and saw that our health and the health of our children is the very core of what is important in life?

What if we all reclaimed our adulthood, decided that we were not going to be led around, that we had the strength to say no, that we could make our own decisions about food—we weren't too rushed, too helpless, too overwhelmed to care about our health? What if we decided that we didn't care —really didn't care— what the neighbors thought about our decision to get off the merry-go-round, to think for ourselves, to place what is really important into the forefront of our daily lives?

What if we really began to see the bigger picture? To operate on the truth that we know in our hearts: that the next generation's lives are dependent on us, that we, as humans, are part of a larger, intricately interwoven system and the decay and destruction of one part affects the entire organism called life. We have been living selfishly for too long. The era of gluttony is over.

The era of seeing ourselves as separate and distinct from –and in competition with— our neighbors is over. The earth under our feet, the water and air around us and in us is a part of us, affects our cells, affects our offspring. The pesticides that caused the thinning of the shells of birds and the disappearance of the bees have parallels in us: autoimmune diseases, cancers, members of our species who suffer from the diseases of "age" in their childhoods: diabetes, high blood pressure, heart disease.

Writes 73 year old avid gardener, Patricia Gothard, to the BBC News, "To each his own, live and let live is great, but when it comes right down to it, destroying the world to have quick big bucks will destroy me too and I do not like that at all."[3]

We are no longer willing to turn a blind eye to the mountain of evidence which suggests that the lifestyle we've been living is sabotaging us at every turn. It's time to look behind the message- to pull back the curtain and reveal the not so benevolent men pulling the strings for their own benefit, hoping to hoodwink all in order to retain their power and wealth.

So what do we do?

What is the answer to our confused tailspin, the mealtime maelstrom, our food-choice dilemma? Where do we turn? Who do we trust?

The answer is so simple you may not believe it. So simple that some of you may not be appropriately impressed. This is the earth-shattering message that needs to be conveyed:

Trust yourself.

You don't have to buy any gizmo, you don't have to join any group, you don't have to follow a particular program, eating plan, or daily ritual. You don't have to dress a certain way, speak a certain way, or wear a hairdo or facial hair in any particular manner. Hats, bonnets, headscarves completely optional. You don't have to weigh, measure or count. You don't have to compare anything with friends or acquaintances, though you may find yourself enjoying shared discoveries.

So who's the new authority? Who's in charge? Who tells you what to eat?

YOU.

Your cells know what they need. Your body *knows* what it needs, it's just been derailed by our society, by corporations, by marketers, by just plain, honest ignorance of what good things are out there because you have not been exposed to real foods.

What you have to do is learn, once again, to trust your body.

Re-familiarize yourself with the sensations of fullness and hunger. Re-learn the recognition of your body's messages. It may not happen quickly, but it will happen.

Remember—advertisers and their corporate sponsors will do anything, say ANYTHING to undermine your faith in yourself, to create doubts. Trust yourself, hold fast to your decisions. Come out of the fog. You will breathe easier. You will sleep better. You may even lose weight.

You don't need someone to tell you what is good for you. You already have that information. You don't need books, articles, advisors, specialists. No one has to tell you that vegetables are good for you or that too much of even a good thing is bad. You know that you can't remain healthy on just meat or just breads or just sodas and candy bars.

In your heart you know that the lifestyles we've been straining to maintain are taking a toll, physically and emotionally. It's time to come clean with yourself. It's ok to grow up. Take a deep breath and prepare to step off the merry-go-round.

CHAPTER 5

Reclaiming our Adulthood

"Do not wait for leaders;
do it alone, person to person."
~ Mother Teresa

"It is never too late to be
what we might have been."
~ George Eliot

This is a clarion call to a new Western culture. Stop being bullied. We have been taught over and over that what we ingest is merely something to stop a hunger pang. Something, usually salty or sweet; its only necessary attribute that it please our taste buds. In this way we are encouraged to eat "baby" food: anything that makes us happy and satisfies our desire for immediate gratification.

For decades we've been encouraged to focus on our appearance as the goal in changing our lifestyles, with detrimental results for both women and men. Somebody is raking in the billions we spend on gyms and pills and diets, while we are dragged through the wringer of repeated gain and loss of weight. Vanity simply cannot be the primary goal for most people, it just doesn't provoke enough passion (thankfully) to sustain the average person.

We have to accept that what we put into our mouths throughout the day is not something of passing inconsequence— the need to fill our bellies as we speed through life to the next important engagement. We know that what we eat constitutes not only the building blocks for every cell in our body but, as a result of what those cells receive, it creates our emotional state, our energy levels, our physical condition, our level of mental acuity, our ability to reproduce and the health of our offspring. It colors our level of enjoyment of life.

We have begun to realize that our diet, our choice of foods, affects not only the duration of our lives, but our very experience of it. It's time for us to act on that.

What we eat plays a major role in our health. It also defines us as a person. Convenience food is not only disastrous for our bodies, it is selfish. It says, "I don't care that these companies are aggressively targeting children and willfully undermining the health of the future generations. I don't care that the laborers at the meatpacking plant that produced this meat are some of the lowest paid and have some of the highest injury rates of any industry in the country. I don't care that the animals used to create this meal lived lives of misery and pain. I don't care that the people in towns all over our country are sickened by the smells and runoff of sewage and chemicals created by the manure lagoons[1] around the factory dairy farms used to make this milk or milkshake."

If we feed convenience food products to our children, it says, "I don't care about the health or future of my own children, all I care about is my own convenience." And it says far more.

We are destroying our planet with our food lifestyle.

Most people do care. They've simply never thought about food in broad terms. Now, nascent awareness of the implications of our choices has shaken many people. As horror stories about every aspect of our ferocious, merciless, greed-driven industrial approach to food production have surfaced over recent years, people have begun to try to find alternatives.

> "The ultimate measure of a man is not where he stands in moments of comfort and convenience, but where he stands at times of challenge and controversy."   ~Martin Luther King, Jr.

We cannot continue to confront nature in the way we have in the past: as if it were a thing to be conquered; against which to test one's self. This is an adolescent approach to nature. This approach evolved quite understandably when you think that most of our human history is a story of conquering untamed wilderness by people who rarely lived past 35 years. We live in a different time.

We have been acting like the young male who feels the need to test boundaries, to fight, or to confront the reigning hierarchy, to prove himself against *something* as he comes of age. We have been striving to rein in, to conquer, to control nature. As a species, we have a difficult time accepting that we are helpless against the unpredictability of forces beyond our understanding. We are counting on the shamans of science to redeem us, absolve us and deliver us from all our foibles, be they dietary or environmental. We somehow believe that no matter what we do, scientists will pull us from the brink of the many disasters we seem to be careening towards.

We cannot control Nature, we never have and we never will. Nature as we know it will unravel before it cedes control to us— therein revealing its trump card because when Nature disintegrates, our species perishes. And then... Nature will come back without us, scarred but resilient.

Instead we have to take a more adult approach to our place in the natural world. We can no more control our surroundings than a cell in a Petri dish can control the medium in which it lives. We have to learn to come to terms with our "Petri dish" and turn our attention, not to escaping earth (throwing ourselves blindly at the edges of space, hoping to find a new planet to populate) or butting heads with Nature, but to living in balance with our world. We must learn to manage and maintain it in such a way that it sustains us.

The new paradigm rewards those who work with, not against our environment. It mythologizes not those who strip-mine the life out of our farm land (or any other land), who slash and burn, who conquer, take and move on, but those who achieve the most with the least: the least disturbance to the soil, the least destruction of the ecosystem, the least pollution of the air and water.

Laws will not be the impetus for the changes in our access to quality food. What we need is for people's understanding of the real repercussions of poor diet to change, for them to start making simple alterations in their food choices. Then move on in action to major changes. People's pride in their health and the health of their children, their level of compassion for livestock animals, their environmental concerns, all have begun shift as we begin to forget the almighty "bottom line" for the sake of doing right in the world.

Unquestionably, there had to be an end to "endless" profit. We are witnessing the inevitable outcome of avarice and short-sightedness in our current global economic turmoil. Until the man who undercuts quality for the sake of unethical profit is recognized not as more clever or more enviable but as despicable and worthy of disdain, we will not have food security. I believe that day is coming when we will willingly move away from the conceits of greed and hedonism.

Many people are worried about the food recalls on the news so regularly. Or are concerned about the wisdom of ingesting the growing inventory of medications we rely on or worse, that are now being prescribed for even our youngest children. One can't help but notice that the latest pharmaceutical industry trend is to encourage us to take daily medications for the rest of our lives for afflictions which we may not yet have and may never have gotten. Furthermore, these are drugs for which the long term effects on other systems in our bodies have not been studied.

You want to do what's right for your health and your family's health and it's begun to occur to you that the messages we're being bombarded with change and contradict one another with disturbing frequency. They often don't seem to make sense. They certainly don't address any long term approach to true wellness. Watching TV it's easy to feel like the naïf in some Dickensian urban alley being lured, cajoled, pawed at and tantalized by lurid characters from up and down the dark street. Everyone's selling you the cure, offering quick riches if you'll follow them. They're all flashing gold and sunshine and dreams. Everyone's telling you they have the answer.

I think you can find the answer in yourself. In Peter Singer and Jim Mason's *The Way We Eat*, MaryAnn, the wife and mother in one of the sample families, chidingly calls her husband Jim a "purist" in his eating habits. Jim rejects most modern fare and sticks with foods raised without chemicals and raised locally. It's a very simple diet. He does the homework and makes his own choices. We may not all make the same choices, but I like that label. It describes exactly what I want my food to be: pure. I want my food free of adulterants and man-made chemicals, free of nano-bits and so-called medication or "enrichment", free of toxic sludge. In fact, I want my air and water and soil that way also. Just the way that nature provided it for me.

I don't pretend to know why we're here or how the earth evolved to feed us as well as all the animals and insects and birds and amphibians. Or how our remains serve to feed the plants, which clean the air and sustain the water. I don't know. But I do know that that's what I want to be a part of. That, in fact, I am a part of the whole. And I want to respect and nurture this intricate system. I don't want the whole thing brought down by the selfishness and carelessness of a few greedy people. Call me a Purist. I am proud to be one.

"You can't cross a chasm with two small jumps."

~David Lloyd George

Go for it. Trust yourself. Anyone can change their eating patterns and buying practices with a new outlook and a willingness to work at it. I will not claim that changing old habits will be easy, convenient or that there's one simple "one-size-fits-all" approach. The good news is that I'm also not going to try to sell you a "magic pill." There is none. We are not children. It is time to roll up your sleeves and face, like an adult, the most important changes you will ever make in your life. We have been taught our entire lives not to trust ourselves. Reflect on that for a moment.

All it takes to begin eating well is a rising anger at the insults and indignities we encounter everyday –the contemptible fodder they are passing off in glossy boxes, the labyrinthine store design to ensure that we see all the things they intend for us to buy, their unconcealed expectation that we can all be led like toddlers, with a cinnamon scent here or a shiny, sparkly, flashing object over there— and a determination to see the whole picture with new eyes. If you haven't yet begun in some measure to seek the path of real health, of freedom from the manipulations of the pharma-agricultural machine, then join us now.

Reclaiming our Adulthood

I am not going to encourage you to write to your congresswoman, petition corporate CEOs, start a phone campaign to the FDA, or carry placards outside of Cargill, Syngenta, ADM, Tyson, Monsanto or any other agribusiness multinational. (Though I'm not discouraging any of these activities, either!) This is not about appealing to the authorities to protect us, this is about protecting ourselves. Only your own actions can safeguard your family and your community.

The days of expecting a benevolent, paternal organization, government, profession, or agency to provide a shielding arm from the onslaughts of life's dangers, well, it was a fairy tale to begin with, a myth. There are people who will demand that our *leadership* has to respond, to take the helm. I say no. We can't wait. *You* must participate. No one is undertaking in a purely altruistic way to take care of you, they are each trying to take care of their own jobs, their own achievements, reputations, and financial security. You must act.

For one thing, we have to stop being distracted. It is a sad truth that most of our media is owned by big business. We are no longer scandalized or even surprised that news is biased. How often do we watch a cheery newscaster exclaim, in one long breath in a 10-second spot, that 99% of all Americans have excessive levels of chemicals in their bloodstream and then without missing a beat move into an equally cheery and effervescent 30-second spot on the latest woes of some addled celebrity? (Then skip to a commercial promoting those very aforementioned chemicals.)

Or a spectacular foul shot will be repeatedly shown and talked about throughout the day, debated excitedly among anchors, while in a tiny strip across the bottom of the screen the real news of corporate takeovers, predatory lending, job losses, usury, and multimillion dollar CEO benefit packages silently flickers. When all stories are given equal weight, we tune them out equally. Worse, some stories never make it through the corporate filters.

We cannot just hop into our four-wheelers or grab our skis or our golf clubs and count on someone else to protect us. You have to become the leader. Each of you have to take charge of your own life and your children's lives. And your food is your life.

Fortunately, it's simple:

- Stop buying decoy foods.

- Don't be sucked in by "Baywatch" fruits and vegetables.

- If it needs a label, you don't really need it.

- Resist the hypnotic enticements of junk food marketing. Don't allow yourself to be distracted by the shiny objects.

- Give up fast food. Are you an "addict?" Start by cutting down to only once a week. After a month, cut back to once a month. After three months, quit. Or get tough and go cold (free-range) turkey.

- Stop filling your days with less significant activities and make the choices that count.

Here's one idea for a new approach: decide to try to avoid eating anything that comes out of plastic. You could call it the "No Plastic Diet." Plastic tubs, plastic containers, plastic bags— unless it's something you made and are storing in your freezer, you will probably be better off without the contents, and you will undoubtedly be better off without the plastic by–products which have leached into the food as well. (Though frozen unadulterated fruits and vegetables would be an obvious exception as far as items in plastic being "allowed" on the "diet." I suspect also that there is far less leaching, if any, when items are frozen.)

In terms of goal-setting, it is important to understand what the temptations will be. Know that you will have to withstand the peer pressure of fast food lunches or the night out at the family-style chain restaurants. Better yet, create other, new gatherings around eating and companionship and have your friends and family join you. Set the example. Decide that you are willing to change your lifestyle and remain firm. Decide to eat simple meals, make choices not because you "have" to but because you choose to, not because the economy is "making you suffer" or "cut back," but because you believe in the choices you're making.

In the words of Aristotle, "We are what we repeatedly do. Excellence, then, is not an act, but a habit."

If each of us, today, decided that we were concerned enough to make the change, that we were willing, for the sake of our children's and our own health, to commit to buying only organic foods for even three months, we could rock the world. Accept the responsibility. Stop blaming the authorities. Stop looking to "daddy" to check your tomatoes before you eat them or to research the chemicals in your coco kringles. Step away from the battle. Make an unwavering commitment to right your own life. You know how.

We are increasingly becoming a two class society~ the rich and the not rich. You may read about pasture-raised pigs and think "those animals live better than some people in my community!" Well, the rich will always have things you don't have, but you don't have to let anyone take your health from you. You might think of organic food as only for the wealthy but consider soft drinks, used pervasively across all economic levels, and conceive this — if everyone, right now, quit drinking soft drinks of ANY kind and spent that extra money on better quality food it would change the course of history. Change is within your grasp, no matter your current financial state.

American consumers spent more than $270 billion for the 36 billion gallons of fountain and packaged beverages they consumed in 2005. That mind-boggling amount is about what American families spent on gasoline that year.[2] In the realm of faux-foods and bad beverages, soft drinks, particularly carbonated, are some of the worst that you can put in your body. Quitting them is a win-win for your health and your pocketbook.

[According to the peer-reviewed journal of the Academy of General Dentistry (AGD), the latest of many recent studies shows that tea, green or black, is a better choice for your health and your teeth.

Green tea, uncarbonated and *without* milk, lemon or sweeteners of any kind, is full of natural antioxidants, which are thought to decrease incidence of cancer, diabetes and heart disease. The study found that the sugars and acids found in both sodas and the fruit drinks that so many parents replace them with, are more erosive to tooth enamel than hydrochloric or sulfuric acid (also known as battery acid.) Find unsweetened tea too bitter? Don't sweeten it, water it down.][3]

Consider these statistics from the Environmental Defense Fund: "If every American skipped one meal of chicken per week and substituted vegetables and grains, for example, the carbon dioxide savings would be the same as taking more than half a million cars off of U.S. roads. And speaking of cars, it takes fuel to transport food, so buying from local farmers and ranchers cuts emissions even if you don't cut out any meat. If every American had one meat-free meal per week, it would be the same (in terms of fuel savings) as taking more than 5 million cars off our roads. Having one meat-free *day* per week would be the same as taking 8 million cars off American roads."[4] Make the unselfish adult choice. Give up your soft drinks. Alter your weekly dinner menu. Be the change.

It is easier to walk a worn path than push through brush, but once a new path is broken it soon becomes comfortable and accustomed while the old way grows over with weeds. It is the same with good habits. Once you begin to really resolve to commit to one small part of a healthy life, the next step comes easier, and the next easier still. Soon you find that you are not as intrigued as you once might have been by the "temptations" and unhealthy choices. A bag of "cheese" puffs or a cappuccino-flavored beverage made from soy oil and high fructose corn syrup, seen from the vantage point of an accountable aware adult perspective, are recognized for what they are: a reckless abomination of chemistry foisted on the foolhardy for the sake of greed. Their tastes become salty sawdust and cloying oil in your mouth.

And what is an adult? I have often seen far more adult behavior in people considered "young adults," that is, thirteen thru twenty, who are, with sincerity and hope, volunteering their spare time at Habitat for Humanity or working in community gardens or another community service, than in many others in their thirties, forties or older who throughout their lives have behaved like selfish five year-olds, stepping on others to accumulate material wealth. Being adult, in the view of this book, is defined by behavior not age. Anyone can act like an adult and begin to take charge of his or her life. I welcome young people with the foresight, courage and conviction to take an adult stance. They will make a difference in the world.

So where do I start?

We boast that food in our culture is seemingly ubiquitous, declaim ourselves the land of plenty. The truth is: it doesn't count if it's not real food. Real food is just as rare as in historical times, the only thing that is ubiquitous is our ability to fill our bellies and placate our hunger with something that tastes acceptable to our downtrodden palate. Many of these "foods" are no more nutritious than the grass and mud ingested by the desperately poor on other continents. Many of them are worse than non-nutritious, they're detrimental. We are paying the price for allowing ourselves to be fooled.

It is not necessary to elaborate the many ways that simple, unadulterated foods will provide you with the things that your body was meant to have, because you know it in your heart. They may be able to fool our eyes, they may be able to trick our sense of smell or seduce our taste buds, but there is one sense that the agribusiness scientists have not been able to fool, not irreparably. Common sense. Common sense may have been sidelined temporarily, we may have pushed it away for the sake of self indulgence, but deep down we still have it and it can't be outsmarted if we choose to listen.

Once we decide to stop playing the games, to stop giving credence to all the external voices encouraging us in different directions and to be completely honest with ourselves, we know exactly which foods are good for us. Nobody has to tell you, once you decide to grow up.

Unpasteurized, un-irradiated, un-chemically-saturated foods

–yes, locally grown, in season, organic foods– are what our bodies were adapted to utilize since the beginning of time. To reiterate an easy guideline: if it has to have a nutrition label, avoid it. Snow peas don't have a nutrition label. Oranges don't have a nutrition label. Rice, potatoes, pork chops, none of these things, whole and unprocessed, require a deciphering of contents.

By locally grown, it is sufficient to consider one's region of the country so that people in urban areas do not have to feel that the food must be grown down the block. An area that is experiencing the same climate as you are at any given time within a reasonable circumference of you can be interpreted to be local. You decide the meaning of reasonable. (If you do it honestly and fairly than you will be eating locally.) A diameter of one hundred miles is taken by many to constitute a local area.

One of the first things to consider when weighing your options in food choices is the long term picture. We have been conditioned for decades to pay attention to only the "now." Immediate gratification is the siren song of the retailer. Maturity looks to the future. "Penny wise, pound foolish," is the cliché, but it remains true. It just doesn't make sense to save a buck or two on a habit of cheap meals to then throw away hundreds on doctors to treat your irritable bowel syndrome gotten as a result of that diet.

For the long term these changes will mean not only that your health will improve but your dependence on OTC and prescription potions and pills will abate or possibly cease entirely. It will also mean, in the long term, that our soils will be improved by increased enrichment with natural amenities, there will be less toxic runoff into our streams and waterways. This translates to less expense incurred to purify our drinking water. It is the start of the rejuvenation of our surroundings, upon which we depend and of which we are an intricate part.

Unfortunately, one of the recurrent themes I have begun to hear on the news channels when discussing our country's recent economic downturn is that people are giving up those "pricey organic foods" and turning to fast food and whatever is inexpensive at some big box store to keep their families fed. The media mantra is "cheap, cheap, cheap." They would have us believe it's our only recourse. Nothing could sound more ridiculous, (unless your sponsor is a fast food or junk food conglomerate.)

Many people are compelled by habit (and perhaps corporate suggestion) to claim that the seeming priceyness of organic foods puts those foods out of the realm of possibility for their daily fare, and here I beg to differ from personal experience.

For more than two decades I have held to what I call "The 90/10 rule." Ninety percent (roughly) of my weekly diet, despite living quite hand-to-mouth for much of that time, consisted of and currently consists of organic foods. I made the choice to allow 10% of my dietary intake to be "other" to enable me to participate in potlucks and picnics, to be a guest at someone's house without being a difficult guest, and to allow for unforeseen incidents. It is a way of participating in social events, family events, restaurant occasions where you will not be able to follow your own new found dedication because of circumstances outside your control.

If your mother-in-law, once in a blue moon, presents you with a pan of homemade sausage lasagna made from the grocery store she's shopped at for 30 years, know that she is well-intentioned. If your co-workers are having a potluck to raise money for a family made homeless by a fire: Eat. If a dish has been made with love, allow yourself some flexibility until the rest of the world catches up. On the other hand, don't cave in to peer pressure. Don't participate in every birthday bash or candy bar fundraiser in the office. Stick to your game plan. Set a quiet example.

I say "roughly" 90/10 because I am not one for measuring, I don't keep charts, or records, I don't beat myself up if I stray; it is merely a guideline. The things I bought, the food I cook at home, was and is organic. But the 90/10 rule really means something close to 90/10, not

50-50. This is where it is most important that you are completely honest with yourself. Heroically and solemnly honest. No one is watching or checking up on you. Food choice becomes a personal spiritual journey. It is a matter of desire and passion, a matter of making the decision to take that untrod path and then doing so with conviction and vision.

One of the impetuses of writing this book has been to demonstrate the need and the possibilities for healthy eating to those who may feel that participation in the healthy eating movement is out of their economic realm. It seems that much of what I've read on the topic of this new direction in food choice has been aimed at those who are far wealthier than I. While I have come to similar conclusions as they and made similar choices, these books, erudite and insightful though they have been, are off-putting to people I've met at the warehouse and service industry jobs that I've had.

It would appear, if one were to rely only on the books and magazines currently available, that healthy food choices are the prerogative of those for whom choices of all kinds are an assumptive condition: which house to summer in, which new hybrid car to buy, the New Alternatives Fund or Portfolio 21 to stash the extra cash? While these other options may not be available to everyone, healthy, organic food certainly is.

In brief: I have never owned a vehicle that has not been third-hand, I do not currently own a home, no less a second home. I do not have health insurance and have only very briefly had it in the past. My health insurance is my health. I protect that with my whole being.

My groceries are nearly all organic or as free from man-made toxins as I can find. A good example of a healthy compromise is cheese. Cheese is expensive and not something I have often. However, when I do purchase it, I only buy imported cheeses from the European Union. They are not organic, per se, but these countries do not allow rBST/BGH or antibiotics to be used on their livestock. In European countries a long history of inviolable cultural traditions and pride in their end products usually ensures that they aren't about to resort to cheap tricks to produce quick shoddy knock-off goods to turn a fast euro.

In contrast, typical American food producers with no comparative history, no reverence, no ties to tradition or "the old way," will often stop at nothing to make a cheaper more "cost effective" product, constrained only by the flimsy laws we have in place that they haven't yet been able to work around. There are completely organic producers in this country whose cheeses I will buy on occasion, but far less in the way of variety of cheeses is being produced.

In my life I have even done an eight month long stint as a cross country truck driver, yet maintained my organic meals with a little ingenuity and perseverance despite being on the road for 4-6 weeks at a time. I was very thorough in my planning when I shopped. I had a little camp stove for cooking my brown rice and a small cast iron pan for sautéing my garlic, onions and other things.

I grew a rotating variety of sprouts in jars in the sleeper of the truck so that I would have some fresh vegetables and always had my water filter filtering water because I didn't like that store-bought sometimes had a plastic-y taste. Cooking my healthy little meals in the truck was the happiest part of the whole adventure for me.

One of the differences, perhaps, between my meals and those of many other people is that I eat very simply. Rice and pasta are my mainstays, with lots of veggies, beans and various sauces. I make a lot of soups, and nearly always bake my own homemade bread. (Not on the road, of course.) Amusingly, people who don't know me have always assumed that I was a vegetarian. I currently raise meat rabbits. Other meat has always been a rare treat because I seek out grass-fed and naturally raised organic meats when I do buy it. (The word organic has been abused, certainly, but I research the food as well as I am able.)

I am very fortunate, at this point in time, to live in a rural area where I am able to grow a large portion of my food in a small garden (400 sq. ft.) and raise a handful of rabbits as well as guineas, chickens and turkeys –which I process myself– so I eat more meat than I ever have before. But this means 3-5 times a week, not 3x a day. Ask any vegetarian, there are countless delightful ways to fix various beans and rice/ corn/ wild rice/ pasta dishes so that one really never has to feel bored or deprived.

Another difference is that I relish leftovers. Sometimes prepared individual things like rice can be made into a different dish the next night, or used for something like rice and eggs in the morning instead of toast –one of my favorites. (Sauté the cooked rice with onions, then break the eggs right into a little "nest". Cook them just over easy, so they're still runny in the middle—if your eggs are from outdoor free-range chickens on a farm with only 20-30 birds, you really don't have to worry about cooking the life out of them for safety's sake. Add a little salt, freshly ground pepper and fresh rosemary and when you eat it, smunch the eggs all around with the rice. Yum!)

Many times a dish really benefits from sitting overnight. Soups and stews and pasta sauces all improve with a little time. I recall in the 1990s being startled and rather disappointed when a friend whose income had recently substantially improved, stated that she never ate anything that was a leftover and "couldn't" eat a piece of bread if it was a day old. This had become a common refrain among the upwardly mobile. All I could think of was the waste. My homemade bread is fine for several days for sandwiches and toast, especially if tossed in the fridge after a day or two. And then, what about French toast, breadcrumbs, bread pudding? She probably threw out more food than she ate. What a shame. We soon lost touch. Martha Rose Shulman on the other hand, writing for the NY Times, has done a whole series of recipes using stale bread. I love her for it.

I usually cook up a large pot of rice and one of beans on Sunday and then fix them in various ways for as long as they last throughout the week. I am perfectly comfortable eating the same exact dish for several days in a row if it's something I like. The next week might go in a different direction, with root vegetables as the base of the meal for a few days, or pastas.

I make a lot of very simple soups to freeze and then take to work for lunches. Right now I work part-time as a baker and on weekends at home I bake my own bread. I've never owned a bread machine. Why take the fun out of it?

I enjoy cooking tremendously and especially when it requires some creative thinking. My sister Diane and I, though we live a thousand miles apart and in wildly different environments— I live in a very rural area, she in the center of Manhattan— have long shared self-invented recipes. Often the recounting of the meal is the sole reason for a phone call, and will begin excitedly with something along the lines of this: "Ok, I opened the fridge and I had a two mangos, some leftover shrimp, a bulb of garlic, a bag of raw peanuts..." And with triumph, the entire stir-fry or casserole or multifaceted meal will be delineated in all its savory detail, concocted of odds and ends and ingenuity.

One of my own favorite personal creations was based on a pasta topping which I typically made with sautéed garlic, pine nuts, minced fresh parsley and sun-dried tomatoes, an Italian classic. Only I was out of sun-dried tomatoes. Here I will confess that I often think of the composition of a meal as akin to working with an orchestra to compose a musical score (not that I have ever composed music, mind you.) All the elements of the orchestra should be available for a well-rounded piece, but each section can be represented by varying instruments depending on the mood and substance of the piece; piccolos might take the place of bells, or violas stand in for French horns.

In this spirit, when I realized that I was out of sun-dried tomatoes as the garlic already simmered, I poked around and hit on a pint of fresh blueberries. Like the dried tomatoes they are very intense in flavor and sweet, yet tart. In the theme of the orchestra I decided this complex flute section could "play" the soulful violin part I was accustomed to. I sautéed them to a gentle softness with the rest of the ingredients and topped my angel hair pasta. It was exquisite. So good, in fact, that I had friends over several nights later and recreated it to their great delight.

The point is that eating well, even eating nearly all organic food, does not have to be expensive and is never boring. In truth it is cheaper to eat the way I do than to buy endless, expensive packaged meals, snack-ables, pre-cut bits of vegetables and just-add-water boxed things. It is far cheaper than eating out when "eating out" consists of real food at a real restaurant, especially with the cost of travel and tip. It is even cheaper than fast food.[5]

The cost of living for a month entirely on a rich variety of fresh, whole, organic foods, including meats when used sparingly in a healthy manner, is no more expensive than a full months worth of low-end prepared processed foods for the same number of people when one puts a little thought into shopping.

Americans spent an average of $1926 per person on groceries in 2007 according to the US Agriculture Department (remember that most American's meals were eaten out during that time period.) In that same year, eating 90% organically and eating out no more than 10 times the entire year, I spent $1958.20, which included several expensive bottles of cod liver oil and a calcium supplement.

Organic brown rice and organic dried beans, purchased in bulk and prepared en masse for the week with spices and greens and whatever else you have on hand, wrapped in a whole wheat tortilla and frozen, costs just pennies, maybe a dollar and a half, compared with a Whopper and fries at more than six dollars (today) including the soft drink which 90% of consumers purchase with their meal.

Don't disdain rice and beans. "Living on rice and beans" is a cliché in our culture synonymous with poverty. But it shouldn't be. Eating organic brown rice, maybe a rare variety, and seeking out exotic organic heirloom beans of some kind could become as much a source of financial flamboyance as eating steak has become, if that's what motivates you. A better choice would be to be driven by the health benefits they would afford you.

Certainly, if you can learn to be motivated by the act of seeking the best, most nutrient dense, lean, healthy choices for yourself and your loved ones, then simple, pure, organic rice and beans of any variety can be seen for what they really are: life-giving, belly-filling, soul-sustaining goodness.

I am dismayed when I hear from people within the "struggling" economic class claim that they cannot afford real food. I feel compelled to explain that it really isn't more expensive, it's part of the long term picture of reclaiming your health, as I have elaborated above. On the other hand, I become irate when I hear this argument from denizens of the middle and upper middle class.

Nothing you do, not one thing, is more important than the food choices you make. Nothing you do for your children, be it piano lessons, private tutors, or paying for the new science building to gain them entrance to your alma mater— is going to be of more consequence in their lives than providing them with real, whole, home-cooked, untainted foods and teaching them why you are doing so, in conversation and by example. We are just beginning to see the tip of the iceberg as regards the long-term health of future generations and the planet they will be living on, and it isn't pretty.

When I recently made a disparaging comment about "American cheese food as a non-food" in front of a friend, he said "Well, it's great for kids, it's cheap and they don't know the difference. It's perfect." (He has two kids.) Nothing could be further from the truth.

The idea of pawning off second-rate goods on the unsuspecting is not new. Throughout history it has been one of the main reasons food oversight laws have been instituted. But the idea that we are now seeing our own offspring as ignorant suckers who can be huckster-ed with impunity is unthinkable.

Beware the websites which offer coupons enticing you to the cheapest food to be had. Some attempt to lure you with the illusion that this "savings" is your goal, "as a Mom." But how do these coupons become available? The companies who make the products provide them. And which products are they providing coupons for? Not what you might want, but the ones *they* want you to buy: the products with the highest return on the dollar for them, made with the cheapest ingredients. A quick glance at one such site brought up coupons for Lucky Charms cereal, 3 or 4 variations on a freezer-tube of sugar-coated white flour rolls, Coffeemate and several more for refrigerated cookie dough. When is the last time you saw a coupon for a head of cabbage? Your kids deserve better.

But my kids won't eat it...

Good or bad, children will eat what they are given —eventually. As battalions of marketers have already discovered, children are a captive audience. But they don't do the shopping, you do. They're not the ones paying for it, you are. The problem is that we have been encouraged —by the marketers— (for several generations now) to let the children have whatever they want. Others have jumped on this bandwagon. Psychologists, psychiatrists and all manner of therapists and advisors have lectured us to give children choices in order to build their autonomy and self esteem. Fine. Let them choose what shoes to wear. When it comes to their food they are not capable of understanding the environmental, physical, medical, social and cultural implications of one product over another. Your children are being led by somebody. Let that somebody be you, not an advertiser.

In close-knit old world cultures, traditions, including eating traditions, were often passed on quite rigidly. This had some advantages and other disadvantages, but no matter. We generally do not live in that kind of environment anymore in the West. However we can learn from their methods and experience to create a new paradigm with the advantages of the old: pride in our own ways, a distilling into our children of the conviction of our choices, a sense of unity within the family and a sense of community with like-minded people. We are free to leave behind any vestiges of things that have been done for reasons no longer remembered.

Thousands of people across this country have begun to do just that. It is the creation of a new community, a movement away from isolation—away from voice recordings and inaccessible faceless CEOs; from untraceable bits of a million different tomatoes hailing from a dozen states and several countries all in one jar of salsa. It is a movement towards buying your tomatoes face to face from Helen, who picked them this morning at her farm and brought them to your local market. If there is a problem with a tomato, you know exactly where it came from. It is a movement towards connection.

Within the United States there have always been numerous small groups of people who do believe enough in their choices that they maintain a separation and isolation from mainstream society despite being surrounded by it. Mennonites, the Amish, Hasidic and Orthodox Jews, devout Muslims, all maintain the observation of laws and rules governing food and often dress which place them at a distance from others in their larger community. Their children are taught the rules, and the reasons for them. If you are not already a member of one of these groups, you can teach your children your rules. What is important is not what the rules are, but your own sincere and undeviating faith in and fulfillment of those rules. You set the example. And you explain, quietly, that "this is what *we* do." It's not a chore, it's a choice.

One parent wrote this comment to a current newspaper columnist's blog on children's health:

> "How do you handle movie dates or meals out where all the other four-year-olds are drinking soda? (And I live in well educated, affluent Montgomery County, Maryland, just outside DC, so it's not like my son's friends' parents are unaware of health and nutrition!)"

The columnist offered suggestions on ways to speak with the other parents, on alternative choices to offer the child (a child will always want what the other children are having, it's not only natural, I believe it's a biological given: animals will exhibit the same behavior), on discussions to have with the child (In my view these discussions are good and should be had with your children from the earliest age, but don't expect results until the child is grown.)

There's actually a very simple answer. Don't go. It is not important that your four-year-old see that particular movie. He will not be damaged by missing a play date –or a dozen play dates. He *will* be damaged by the introduction to a lifetime of the casual acceptance of carbonated beverages as social status quo. As he gets older he will go out on his own and probably encounter all manner of things you would rather he didn't. He will experiment. But your thoughtfully communicated guidelines in his early years will help to govern his positive choices in later life.

One time, in the past, my sister hooked me up with a job she was doing at a huge medical convention during her brief employment with an advertising agency. We were to man a booth in which we lured doctors, with the promise of a t-shirt, to answer a survey regarding which pharmaceuticals they used and why. It was a remarkable experience to watch six-figure salaried professionals quibbling over a t-shirt, but even more unforgettable was the booth next door. They were selling pediatric playroom accessories. Countless parents parked their children with the ill-fated sales folk and left to wile the afternoon covetously stockpiling t-shirts and keyrings, mousepads and little flashlights. They would then return and, kneeling, ask little Angelina or Broderick if it was time to go yet.

Invariably the child would wail "NO" and the parent would retreat to give the little tyke more play time until, after cajoling and imploring, they'd ask repeatedly, "couldn't we please go soon??" The child eventually acquiesced. Some parents were there waiting for more than an hour. Only one couple, from India, walked up and simply picked up their child.

The child screamed and protested—for about the length of half an aisle— while the father, ignoring the screams as he carried the boy, patted him gently on the back and walked on. It was over as quickly as it started. In the meantime, little Mackenzie and Naomi and Wentworth continued to bounce and grab and jostle on the playsets while their parents checked their fancy watches and looked on forlornly.

Don't be that parent. Your children are your wards, not your peers. They don't tell you what they eat, you tell them. Don't kowtow to members of your family who balk at real food, teach them with patience and persistence. Teach your children that you have to feed them correctly, even if they don't like it—it's your job, your responsibility as a adult. We don't always like our obligations. But there can be a sense of satisfaction and empowerment when we meet those demands head on.

It is so necessary that today's children have a chance to learn this. We can no longer—as recent generations had hoped to do—go through life shirking and avoiding the difficult things, and trying to fill our every moment with only fun. The result has been that the *fun* feels empty. It is not a reward, just a filler until the next fun.

Our lives feel shallow and devoid of meaning without responsibility. We bounce like hapless pinballs from one captivating activity to the next seeking a fulfillment that never arrives. Each generation is more wound-up and unfocused than the last.

Give your children the gift of responsibility by instilling in them the self-respect of healthy eating. Food is not supposed to be a plaything. Our children have enough toys. Give your child the satisfaction and self-confidence of knowing what is good for them. Teach them the pride of a sense of duty to one's self. Foster an *attitude of gratitude*.

This means restoring a time for silence before eating, a time perhaps for hand-holding, a time for overt thankfulness for the food before everyone. (This could be to Mother Nature, to your god, or maybe even to each other if the fare is something you've worked together to raise.) Above all, give them good health by insisting on healthy meals.

This is not a debate on childrearing practices, it is about food. Your child's temperament, her ability to focus in school, her level of wellness and level of activity, her ability to work, to grow, to one day procreate, all are determined in measure by the quality of her meals now. You cannot afford to get this one wrong.

As important as choosing the right foods for your child is teaching him how to concoct meals from those foods. On the one hand parents seem to complain that there isn't time to fix a healthy meal, while also lamenting the lack of quality time with the kids. The problem is that we see the two as mutually exclusive. I say many hands make light work. The kids should be a part of the food making process. Involve your kids in the preparation.

Do not involve them in the decisions about *what* foods will be eaten (unless the choice is on the order of tomatoes vs. tomatillos, onions vs. leeks, zucchini or yellow squash—and not in the store, but in the kitchen where you already have them,) but in the creation of the meal. Boys as well as girls are fascinated by the seemingly inscrutable science through which some brittle noodles, a lump of pink ground meat and a few other ingredients becomes a delectable lasagna.

Children really do want to learn what the adult world is all about, it is the great mystery of their existence. You are their conduit to that larger world. They want to spend time with you as long as they aren't being browbeaten. And they are more than willing to accept that you may not know how to cook but that you are willing to share the humor of your failures as well as the insight of your experience.

What better way to spend time with your child than in creating delicious memories from the wonderful aromas of the oven or stovetop? The scent of sizzling garlic in a warm kitchen has conjured far more nostalgia than a madeleine.

Pick one day a week to make blueberry muffins from scratch during berry season. Grow a pot of oregano on the windowsill and use it to make incredible homemade pizzas. Let a portion of a potato grow roots and plant it in a bucket of dirt (poke holes in the bottom) and grow a few of your own potatoes. Involve children from the earliest age.

If you are concerned that a sharp knife might be too dangerous for your six year old, consider that in many parts of the world a six year old is already wielding a machete in the labor of the fields. I'm sure that your child, of average intelligence or better, is not less skilled or capable than that child. Patient oversight will foster security and confidence. You also may find that a healthy diet devoid of soft drinks and added sugars will present you with a calmer more attentive child.

Cooking is wonderfully multidisciplinary with very little effort. Where did this eggplant come from? How is cheese made? (Try making some simple farmer's cheese, no equipment necessary!) What culture had a corn god? What do the names of the different pastas mean? [6]

Tip:

Pasta	Translation
cannelloni	little tubes
fettuccine	little ribbons
linguine	little tongues
manicotti	pipes
mostaccioli	little mustaches
orecchiette	little ears
ravioli	little turnips
rigatoni	little stripes
spaghetti	strings
vermicelli	little worms

What does it mean to cut something into quarters? How many ounces in a cup? What kinds of foods did our great grandmother eat and why? The learning possibilities really are endless.

In my experience teaching urban children of all ages to make cheese from fresh goat's milk at Heifer Ranch, I found they were universally enthralled and eager to not only add the vinegar and stir the pot, but willing to drink the whey and try the resulting cheese. The thrill of experimentation can open all kinds of new doors. Of course, the further you can get the child from the television set, with its preached preferences and clichéd dislikes, the easier your job will be.

In this same vein, it is also important to know what your child is being given to eat in school. According to Ann Cooper, the Renegade Lunch Lady, a typical "reimbursable school lunch meal" consists of chicken nuggets, tater tots, chocolate milk, fruit cocktail in HFCS. "That's what the USDA, our government, says is ok for your kids to eat," she says.

She tells us that in 2006 school cafeterias had "$2.40 per day to spend on each kid -- 70 percent of which goes to payroll and overhead. That leaves 72 cents to spend on ingredients." [7] As of 2008 it is $2.57, still less than a latte at your favorite coffee bar in that year.[8]

In 2002, the Physicians Committee for Responsible Medicine (PCRM) launched an ad campaign which called high-fat, high-cholesterol school lunches "weapons of mass destruction." The U.S. Department of Agriculture (USDA) was cited for "putting industry interests before public health by buying up surplus pork, beef, cheese, and other products and dumping them into the National School Lunch Program." [9]

If your children are buying their lunches outside the cafeteria menu, chances are they're not fairing any better. According to Eric Schlosser in *Fast Food Nation*, the American School Food Service Association estimates that nearly a third of public high schools serve "branded fast food," from Taco Bell to Pizza Hut.[10] In 2005, vending machines were found in 17% of elementary schools, 82% of middle schools and 97% of high schools.[11]

Since then there is a fledgling movement at work to get corporate interests out of our nation's schools and see that health-promoting foods are presented to our youth. If you have school age children, you can only win by getting involved.

But my husband won't eat it...

Let me be clear that I am in no way suggesting in any part of this book that women should be the sole provider of meals and protector of the family health in addition to the many other roles they are expected to take on including, for many, full-time employment outside the home.

The perception that women have always been and should therefore be the keeper of the hearth (or in modern times, the stovetop) and that perhaps a return to the era of "mom" in the kitchen will return wholesome goodness to our lives is another product of the industry-driven compartmentalism of our lives.

Reclaiming our Adulthood

Cooking is a pleasure which no one should be denied.

... no Yoga exercise, no hour of meditation ... will leave you emptier of bad thoughts than this homely ceremony of making bread. ~M.F.K Fisher, The Art of Eating

The saddest message Western culture has currently adopted is that cooking is a burden, a chore and something to be hastened through. Some retrograde, hierarchically rigid groups go so far as to see it as the obligation of an obedient woman in her role as servant of her husband. How could it not be seen as a chore under those circumstances? The distressing result of this mindset leaves men and boys excluded from the delights and empowerment of meal-making, as well as creating something that "modern" women dread.

An unbiased glance at history will reveal that gender roles regarding food and drink have made the usual swings from one side to the other and back depending on many cultural factors. Women may have been the inventors of bread and are recorded as being the masters of both baking and brewing, (considered one vocation) in ancient history, but baking became a male art when guilds were common. Later, industrial baking was almost exclusively a male domain, while conversely in the popular mind baking was still considered a woman's skill. With the current focus on a revival of craftsmanship and artisanal baking, female bakers are again emerging as leaders in the profession.

The pursuit of brewing, while still done by women during many early eras, shifted to monasteries in numerous parts of Europe in later times. In today's renaissance of craft brewers, the enthusiasts are nearly all male. Cheese-making is a craft which was notable in being undertaken by both sexes until the age of mechanization when it became, for decades, the province of men. However the rise of artisan cheeses in the US and its emphasis on creativity and quality, is bringing increasing numbers of women back to the fore as artisan cheese-makers.[12]

Likewise the delights of cooking are being rediscovered by some men. Men have always been interested and involved in cooking. It is commonly recognized that nearly all "the great chefs" have been men (women, of course, were not allowed to participate professionally) while simultaneously overlooked that these men had to have arisen from a vast pool of competitors, also male. In numerous cultures past it was unremarkable and presumed that men had a role in the making of meals.

Grace Young, in *Wok Hay: The Breath of a Wok*, provides a beautiful description of her introduction by her father to the secrets of cooking:

> "In fact, the only time I felt completely Chinese was at the dinner table, eating the wonderful Cantonese home-style meals my parents prepared. Mama and Baba (father) were extraordinary cooks and whether we were dining in a restaurant or eating at home, they provided an ongoing commentary on the fine points of Chinese cuisine. Paramount was an appreciation for what the Cantonese refer to as wok hay, the prized, seared taste of food that's been properly stir-fried in a wok.
>
> My father explained that wok hay is achieved when a chef heats a wok until nearly red hot so that a stir-fry cooks in a matter of seconds. As a child I imagined wok hay to be literally the wok's fiery breath imparting a special life force into the food.
>
> As my parents, aunties, and uncles instructed me and shared their recipes, their kitchens filled not only with fragrant and reminiscent aromas, but also with their wonderful stories of life in China."

"You can take my word for it that a yen to cook is in the same rugged tradition as jousting or going on a crusade to fight the Saracens" boasted Victor Bergeron founder of Trader Vic's restaurants.[13]

The book "Cajun Men Cook"[14] states that "In this culinary tradition, there are as many styles of food preparation as there are individual cooks and, in Acadiana, everyone is an excellent cook. But, of course, men and women, generally tend to cook differently, and in different venues. (Men) cook because they love good food, but also because they love the camaraderie, the good times, and the story telling that inevitably accompany meals. Whether preparing blackened redfish, crawfish, shrimp, gumbo, jambalaya, boudin, etouffee, crabs, oysters, sausage on the bayou, or barbecuing a suckling pig on the patio (where cooking time is often gauged by the amount of beer in the cooler), Cajun men have an innate talent for creating taste treats that frequently evolve into legendary culinary delights."

An Eastern European website[15] brags that "Uzbek men have good cooking skills, and chaikhana is the place where they get together and cook pilaw (rice with meat and vegetables) or kazan kabob (fried meat with potatoes). Uzbek pilaf is a very solemn food. It can be considered as an everyday dish as well as a dish for solemn and great events like weddings, parties and holidays. However, locals believe that the best pilaf is always prepared by a man!"

Not long ago, Diario La Estrella, a daily newspaper in Dallas, featured chef Harry Salazar, star of the nationally televised cooking show — Sazonando con Harry— for "his inspirational success story and the opportunity to dispel the myth that Mexican men stay out of the kitchen." Elaine Louie, in an article titled *Tamales Are Hot, As in Popular*, NY Times Style section,[16] tells us that "Once, making tamales was a communal event, with the whole family filling and wrapping, telling stories and singing songs. There is even a word for it in Spanish, tamalada." "If you've never tried making tamales," shares the *Homesick Texan* on her blog,[17] "this is a food rooted in fellowship; doing it alone is not only counter-productive but sorely lacking in fun. Rally your friends and family and get ready for not only a memorable meal but a whole lot of communal joy."

The responsibility for preparing and cooking food throughout Polynesia always fell to the men, according to the Polynesian Cultural Center's webpage.[18] Sage, a commenter to a blog, notes:

> "My ancestors in Hawaii did things rather differently (than current US tradition) - the men were the only ones allowed to cook! Cooking was a spiritual thing the men did. My grandmother, born and raised in Hawaii, can't cook for anything - her three sons take care of all the meals for her, as she expects them to. Ha! I forgot to mention - in the Hawaiian culture I've been raised with, the art of

cooking is very spiritual.

When you feed someone you are giving them a deep gift, something more than a mere trinket - you're giving them life sustaining material! ... Cooking for the family, someone specific, or for yourself is all looked at in my house as acts of love. The cook, whoever they may be (usually myself or my Dad), is viewed as a generous nurturer."

(Good to see that she is breaking the tradition which disallows women the pleasure of working with food.)

It's a shame that modern Western society, with pressure from media, has colluded to try to deprive men or women of the fun, the camaraderie and the delectable taste of success that competency in the kitchen can bring because once this creativity has been unleashed, it is a natural progression to quality ingredients and ever more complicated tastes and flavors. The possibilities for experimentation are endless. The result is self-assurance, creativity, and the gift of a great meal. No one derives gratification, empowerment or triumph from opening a package and throwing it in the microwave. No one is nurtured by peeling the plastic wrap from a Styrofoam tray.

In the U.S., in urban African-American communities an amazing concept called "Real Men Cook" has begun to address this loss. In eleven different cities last Father's Day, a "family tradition that pays tribute to the family" celebrated another year of boys and men sharing the satisfaction of cooking together. The stated goal of the sponsor organization, Real Men Charities, Inc., is to "point up the value and contribution of the males to healthy families and communities."

In other urban circles, at least in the upscale musicians-&-artists circles which form my sister's group of friends, the men-can't-cook mentality has also changed dramatically. This indicative snippet of conversation with Dara Torres (recent silver medalist in the Beijing Olympics) about her partner, David, came from Women's Health Magazine:

What was it about him that won you over?

...I think we have a very good balance -- he's more on the nerdy, low-key side, while I'm energetic. He comes home after working 10 hours, and not only does he cook, he likes to clean up, too, so he can de-stress. I'm like, Go for it![19]

It is commonly the men in these modern relationships who have been attracted to the creativity of cooking and who relish the relaxing routine and the nurturing and decision-making which goes into the family meal planning. Often it appears that the woman, in her 20's–40's and usually active in a career outside the home, is understandably fearful of the claustrophobia of homemaking which limited a woman's participation in the larger world in the era of her mother. Sadly, she has become the one who lacks the skill to whip something up with confidence and aplomb. I say sadly because this sentiment of disinterest is a manufactured sentiment, fostered by those who would prefer that we scarf the prepared and packaged food-like goods they make available.

While certainly not everyone can be expected to follow the same avocation or pursuits, for any human being to not have an interest in their food seems a pathology in itself. Food is what we are and how we continue to exist. There isn't a species on the planet that doesn't spend a significant portion of its day acquiring and eating food. Humans have historically been no different. Industrialization and marketing has changed that dynamic and they tell us it's for the better, but we are not happier and we are certainly not healthier.

Despite the budding interest of urban men finding fulfillment and relaxation in culinary skills, much of the fanfare around buying and preparing food in suburban-American homes and its imagery in the media, still revolves around the female head of household. This is due, in part, to the 1950's hangover-mentality of mom in an apron in the kitchen all day.

Yet, in suburban America the actual phenomenon of working women with stovetop phobias married to culturally circumscribed men has created a world where no one can cook and most, if not all meals are eaten out or bought already prepared. All day grazing has become routine. Boxed breakfasts and heat & serve lunches and dinners are the norm. While this is seen as a formidable success by the makers of expensive, nutritionless snacks and meals, it is a tragedy for men, for women, and especially for their children who will never know the casual banter and warmly shared memories that exemplified the preparation of one's sustenance throughout the rest of history. This can change in middle America as it has begun to change in urban America.

Living as I do in a rural area, I know that there are many men who are excited about being engaged in their children's lives, in contrast to previous generation's expectations of men. There is a pride in passing on the skills of the outdoorsman. It is not a leap for this kind of involvement to include baking bread or cooking meals. As we've noted, there is considerable cultural precedent worldwide.

Finally, there is the simple realization that cooking is not any different from fishing or hunting if one's goals are to pass on survival skills and to spend quality time together. What is more an act of survival than cooking and eating? Any decent mountain man of old knew how to make a good sourdough bread, knew how to preserve vegetables, cook stews and to make jams of the berries he'd picked. In teaching your sons and daughters to cook, you protect them from the shysters who are out there hoping to prey on their ignorance about feeding themselves by selling them less than quality goods. You give them knowledge about really taking care of themselves. What better bonding experience than to learn together? Some men are finding out that, at the very least, it's an incentive to play with a good set of very sharp knives.

The time has come to bring yourself and your family back to health. Eating unpoisoned fare is the only thing that makes sense. Eating organically is simple and doable. Others just like you are already doing it.

CHAPTER 6

Kshamavaani [1]

*Truly, the greatest gift you have to give
is that of your own self-transformation.*
~ Lao Tzu

This is not about changing one minor detail of your life. Despite Western culture's attempts to downplay its significance, food will always retain profound importance in our lives. Food is comfort and nurture. Food is our connection with our ancestry and our family or an example of our willingness to step outside the lines and experiment with new people and ideas. Food is history, celebration, the sharing of love. Food is an irrevocable thread connecting us to the environment regardless of the many layers of metamorphosis it often undergoes.

In terms of frequency food is the one purchase we make more than any other by orders of magnitude. Food is possibly the one thing we think about more than any other if we consider that for most people meals are undertaken two to three times a day. There are the before-meal considerations of what to have, how to make it if you're making it, where to get ingredients, where to get prepared food if you are not making it, how long it will take to fix or drive to, how long it will take to eat it, how much it costs. And that's all prior to the time spent consuming it.

For all these reasons it is not enough to think "This is important, I'll try to think about this stuff the next time I go shopping." The change must be integrated into every aspect of your life until the choice of healthy living, healthy eating and caring for the source of our food –the planet– becomes as intuitive as breathing. All of these are indivisibly constituent to the whole.

As you recycle, you are saving a plot of soil from becoming a landfill, soil that could someday be used for growing food or returned to its natural ecosystem to reduce carbon and increase oxygen to the atmosphere. As you choose organic meat for the health of your children, you are saving a stream from the runoff of a Concentrated

Animal Feeding Operation (CAFO), and you are saving the fish and aquatic life within that stream.

Inversely, according to the Center for Food Safety "every time you flush your toilet or clean a paintbrush in your sink," you may be unwittingly contributing to the toxic sewage sludge in our wastewater which is then used as fertilizer to grow your food.[2] Each choice we make has a consequence larger than ourselves, always.

This chapter's heading is a word you may not be familiar with. Kshamavaani is the name of a holiday in the Jainist tradition. Literally, it means Day of Forgiveness. The purpose of this book is not to incite you to anger any more than is necessary to jog you from complacency and into a commitment to change the world.

Yes, things have spiraled out of control on farms and in pharmaceutical labs, in CAFOs and cafeterias; your own grocery store has become a source of alluring deceits. Our rivers are poisoned, our air is foul. It is natural to feel threatened and angry, to want to compose impassioned letters to companies, to form protests and have marches. It isn't necessary. Just as the Jains practice overt forgiveness as a necessary first step to their own salvation and liberation, we can learn to move beyond the anger of feeling cheated and put it behind us. Our focus is on moving forward. This is our time of Kshamavaani.

The saying goes "A butterfly in China beats its wings, and a hurricane forms in the Atlantic Ocean." We can achieve far more than the result of any one afternoon's protest march by making many small changes in our own lives and committing to them for good. A lone voice quietly demands "organic vegetables or nothing" regarding her eating choices throughout the day.

Day after day, month after month, in time this becomes a tsunami of voices as the strength of her conviction reverberates through those she touches. The consumer who thinks "if they don't have the things I want, I won't buy anything" shakes the industrial-agricultural conglomerate at its foundation. They have long been counting on you to settle for less.

Kshamavaani

With that in mind, your first steps must be taken on many fronts at once. You may want to go through your cupboards right now and discard packages of "breakfast pastries" and sugared cereals, toss the tasteless packaged meals from your fridge. You might resolve to bring a homemade lunch to work tomorrow.

You are aspiring in your change, not just to forgo the office birthday cake but to reach the point where someone offering you a commercial cupcake, for instance, gives you pause. You conjure up the dry bland texture of a chocolate-colored sponge which doesn't taste at all like chocolate, the gritty-sweet waxy oily-ness of its frosting, the utter lack of any real perceivable flavor aside from a sickly-sweetness which leaves a sour taste in your mouth as soon as you've finished it, and you realize that, no, you really *don't* want it. These changes will come.

Your palate, regularly exposed to the complex nuances of apples and strawberries, whole grains and an enticing variety of vegetables will soon recognize, perhaps to your surprise, the natural sweetness of fresh garden carrots or peas, just picked from the vine. You will come to prefer real food as your body rejoices in its rightful course. It will happen over time.

The plan

Sometimes looking at the world with new eyes can feel overwhelming. It might help to have a notebook or even just sit down at the computer or with a piece of paper draw up a plan. Compose a new grocery shopping list focusing on only organic foods. Decide what the week's meals will be, leaving room for leftovers and re-purposing of dishes, made exclusively from healthy, whole foods.

Discuss with your partner and /or children the changes that will be made, and why. Find a place for their involvement. A little bit of preparation beforehand for their questions and possible objections will leave you in a better position to win them over. Determine what night might be the best for a weekly no-meat meal. You may have to start with proclaiming the evening meal a sacrosanct time of togetherness.

This is the difference between changing your diet and changing your life.

A good place to start in changing your life is to involve others. Just as a scheduled walking or exercise program has been shown to be more easily maintained with a partner, so it is for of many of life's endeavors. It is a sad truth of Western culture that we often function in isolation as we hurry through our tasks throughout our day. Our ancestors did not.

As director of the Cottage Industry Program at Heifer Ranch, I taught adults as well as children. And in addition to making cheese as I've already mentioned, I taught Old World skills like carding wool, and candle-making. Invariably, in my adult classes of mostly women, there arose the issue of what our culture perceives to be the tedium of many Old World tasks. Women's chores: shelling enough beans for a family of seven, coring apples for gallons of cider and vinegar, carding wool for hours, these seem incredibly boring to today's mind.

What isn't typically realized is that these activities weren't done in the context of the oppressive solitude that our society sees as the norm. No one was sitting in a cubicle. Rarely, and only under unusual circumstances was anyone in an empty house. Vast, friendless, windswept acres are a peculiar iconology of the American pioneer. They reverberate with us because they were so dismal. And they were remarkable because they were relatively rare. Diaries from the occupants of those tiny cabins express heartbreaking loneliness. Even the pioneers built near to one another whenever possible. Homo sapiens is a pack animal.

Historically, most of human activity was done in community. Many early tribes around the world lived under one roof. In small villages, homes were clustered. Neighbors gathered for nearly every activity. Sisters and mothers and aunts often lived in the same house. Children played in a corner of the room. Or right underfoot. Or participated in the "adult" activities. Basket weaving, candle-making, wine-stomping, even planting, tending fields and harvesting— all these things were done in the company of others. As chapter four showed, in "the old country" meals were often not only put together with the help of one's extended family, but with friends and neighbors. Songs were created, stories shared, advice passed on. Camaraderie is the human condition.

Investigate who within your circle would also be interested in letting go of the urgency and trappings of conspicuous consumption. Who might benefit by trying to wean their dependence on pharmaceuticals, get more exercise, try new foods? Is it a neighbor? A friend from your church or book club? Your daughter or son? All of the above together? The cornerstone of this new movement is community. No more divide and conquer.

It is essential that we share what we've discovered and find out what others are doing. And it's just so much more fun to shop with an enthusiastic companion, to share meal prep as a time of togetherness, even to eat meals with like-minded friends and family. There are many resources online these days to help you to discover things that may be happening right in your own town. Grab a buddy (or two! Carpool!) and head to the market, finding sources of healthy food in your own area.

Remember that a company beholden to stockholders has only one objective, to increase profits. (In fact, our entire economic system is predicated on the conviction that there is a world in which profits can increase quarterly without end, and we have begun to see the foolishness of this attitude.) Bear this in mind when you choose where to shop. Any business where distant people are investing cash and expecting dividends is going to have far less integrity than a place where local people are investing time and cultivating food for their own table as well as yours.

Your best starting point for quality food is to seek out a farmer's market or a local food cooperative. A cooperative is inherently a community-based retail outlet. You purchase a membership, usually offered on a pro-rated multi-year payment plan. For instance, my local food co-op currently charges $20 a year for seven years. Having begun payment, I am entitled to full membership which includes numerous sales and specially discounted items. At the end of that time I stop paying but retain full membership.

The best part is that each member can be as involved as they would like to be, so that, unlike privately owned, or corporately owned stores, if there is a policy you disagree with or some changes you'd like to see made, there is the real possibility of those changes being made because you have the opportunity to directly participate. And yet, there is no obligation to participate. Or even to become a member if you don't care about receiving the discounts or contributing input. You can still buy there.

I have participated in co-ops around the country for 30 years. While I may not agree with all the politics or decisions different groups have made, in my experience across the board they are run by a small group of very dedicated, principled people who, ultimately, are seeking superior quality products for their own families and family networks.

Keep in mind, however, that each group has different purchasing guidelines, voted on and periodically revised by membership. Members make the rules, so while one co-op may not offer ANY products with refined white sugars or HFCS, others might. Some co-ops may not sell meat products. Some co-ops sell wine and beer and others choose not to. As always, it is important to make the tiny effort required to assure yourself that you are in the know. Read their brochure. Ask questions of management. Attend a meeting.

Unlike places such as Walmart where I've been told "they just send us stuff, we can't request anything" and where you know that local management is 50 layers removed from policymakers, where buyers may live in another state and product lines are decided by profit margins, coops exist through your input. They usually strive to hire a small group of knowledgeable staff who share many of your interests in healthy food and chemical-free agriculture.

This does not mean that everything sold at co-ops or at health food stores is healthy for you. Don't think, once you've entered a "healthy" food store, that you don't have to think anymore. Never turn off your brain.

There are far too many unnecessarily sugared cereals (sometimes it's hard to find ones without added sugars), aisles of candy, chips, frozen treats and processed goods. There are marketers lurking at co-ops and health food stores these days, with wholesome "farm country" logos and sincere sounding gibberish labels. Avoidance of processed foods is always a healthier choice regardless of the retail outlet.

Learn to see through some of the ad-hype. For instance "dehydrated cane juice" is sugar, plain and simple. Some will insist that it contains more "minerals and elements of the whole plant" than refined white sugar. Who cares? It's something which should so negligible a part of your diet in any case that eating it with the "added minerals" would not have any benefit whatsoever. Remember, "treats" should not be part of "normal" eating habits. At all. They should be reserved for special occasions, that's what makes them treats. Do not become complacent because someone is telling you their product is good for you. There is no need to be paranoid, but we can no longer be trusting innocents. A savvy wariness is the hallmark of wisdom.

Farmer's markets are also a source of knowledgeable people with an interest in food. However, as I discussed in chapter one, it is extremely important to discuss with your vendor their views and practices regarding use of chemicals. Do not assume because something comes from a winsome booth with baskets of vegetables displayed on pretty fabric that it is necessarily wholesome and good for you. "Homemade" baked goods are often still full of sugar, probably margarine and white flour, even if made in a certified kitchen. They might even be made from a box. Some markets may allow vendors to sell products which they have not grown themselves (most don't.) This would allow someone to buy wholesale from any venue and simply sell them to you at an increased price with a bit of window dressing. It happens. Ask questions.

I have not yet encountered an outdoor market which limits itself to only organically grown produce. Yet many consumers purchase from markets all over the country believing that the food is free from pesticides simply because it comes from a local farmer. This is a huge misjudgment. The word organic has become complex legally, but it is not impossible to understand. It means grown or raised without the use of synthetic chemicals, genetically-engineered seed, sewage sludge as fertilizer, irradiation of the product before it arrives to you, or, as regards animals: use of confinement, antibiotics or hormones.

If "organic" has lost its meaning, think "pure." As discussed earlier, your neighborhood market gardener is as prone as any farmer to use, and even wantonly abuse without any regulation, dicey and dangerous chemicals readily available from their local Ace Hardware or Garden Center. Don't assume anything. As with commercial manufacturers, don't be mislead by façade. A straw hat, Amish bonnet, overalls, flowing skirts and hippie sandals, even a vendor's charming personality—none of these things promise untainted produce or meats. Ask, it's the only way you'll get a sense of the proprietor's beliefs and practices. Typical questions might include:

Do you use any kind of chemicals on your farm/ garden at any time of year? (I've had people assure me their produce was organic because, "We only spray at the beginning of the season." Or that their apples were organic because, "We don't spray the apples, only the tree." These are gross misconceptions.)

How do you deal with insects? (If they insist they don't spray, you may find that they are treating the *soil* with chemicals, or using GE seeds.)

How do you keep the critters (or insert your own word) from your crops? (Rabbits, deer, armadillos, gophers, moles, voles, rats, and other creatures all want a share in the grand buffet of any garden or farm they encounter.)

Do you use organic seed? (A lot of seed is "Round-Up Ready" or otherwise genetically engineered these days. This means that the Round-Up receptive gene is already in every cell of the seed and ultimately the plant it produces.)

If you are purchasing raw milk (cow or goat) you want to be sure that the animals haven't been wormed recently. You also want to know that they aren't being given antibiotics. This would include not only antibiotics which the farmer may administer, but which may already be in their food when it arrives in pellets. Be sure to ask the farmer what they are feeding the cow or goat and if the *feed* contains antibiotics, steroids or other growth enhancers. If the farm claims the cattle are grass-fed, be sure that means 100% of its diet, during all of its life.

There are unscrupulous people everywhere. The growing movement of people who seek healthy food but are unaccustomed to asking questions about that food's pedigree has created a vacuum into which an inevitable contingent of the unprincipled are drawn. I knew a couple who touted their own close ties to a large environmental NGO in marketing their "grass fed" cattle.

Their business was actually a very separate entity. They gave passive customers a false security in believing that the beef was different from the beef of the industrial-agricultural complex. I toured their grounds and asked questions, only to find that their cattle were shipped off at the usual six months of age or so, and "finished" on conventional GE corn-based feed. This is the same dietary regimen a CAFO animal suffers. I was upset that this young couple was selling extremely high priced meat at farmer's markets and through their website under the pretense of "grass fed" because there was no legal definition (at the time) of the term and because their known association with an international organization espousing sustainability caused people to rest on their assumptions. "Grass fed" should mean more than just "my cow has eaten grass."

This kind of behavior has caused consumers to demand change. As of Nov. 15, 2007, the term "grass fed" must mean, by law, that the animal has been fed only grass throughout its life. However, this still does not mean that the grass was grown without pesticides or that the animal even spent time in a pasture. The law does not define the conditions under which the animal must be raised, only what it can be fed. Confined animal operations, in which a caged animal is fed grasses instead of grains, is still legally possible with a "grass fed" label at this time.

You have to decide which concerns are most important to you. If you want to be sure the animal is 100% grass fed *and* raised in pasture that has not been treated with pesticides, that it was not given hormones or antibiotics *and* was allowed to mature in its own time (these are the best possible conditions for your health and the health of the land,) then you have to ask.

Asking questions does not have to feel like an interrogation. You are concerned. A vendor doing the utmost to sell pure unadulterated products wants people to know about it and will appreciate having the opportunity to share with you.

Finally, shop simply. Try to limit yourself to vegetables that are in season. Try to find foods that are grown, raised or produced locally. But first and foremost, be sure that the foods you choose are raised without synthetic chemicals and fertilizers.

For many, this might seem a controversial directive. In the new food movement much emphasis has been placed on carbon miles. "Carbon miles" refers to various ways of assessing the environmental impact of foods by tallying the carbon emissions used in their transportation. Foods that arrive out of season or from out of your area for any reason obviously have accumulated lots of carbon miles. Carbon miles are an important consideration if you are concerned about fuel consumption, depleted oil reserves, smog, ozone holes and climate change; as well you should be.

The focus of this book, however, is your health and the health of our planet. While the health of our planet is certainly affected by all of the above, I feel that by choosing foods that are first and foremost grown or raised without synthetic chemicals, foods that are certified organic (if from afar), (or if local, known to be free of chemicals,) then you have made the best choice for your health, your family's health and for the piece of earth they were grown in or raised on. And since chemical fertilizers and pesticides are synthesized from crude oil, by not using them you have saved that much oil from being depleted.

Additionally, you saved that which would have been used in the ships and trucks which transport the pesticides and fertilizers, the machinery used to create the pesticides and fertilizers, and the petroleum used in their application by tractors, sprayers and airplanes, all belching carbon emissions. You've also spared surrounding rivers and water tables from chemical runoff, beneficial insects including honeybees from poisoning, and the soil from nutrient depletion and toxic accumulations.

If you can also get most of those foods locally, and your food does not have to be wrapped in plastic for storage or shelf life, then you've also saved the environment from the creation of more plastic (another petroleum product of course) and its endless disposal issues.

So, start at your local market by filling your canvas bags (brought from home) with things you already know and like, only the organic version. And here's an thought: on each trip be sure to include something you have never tried before. Health food stores and co-ops have been catering to those who favor the exotic for decades. Remember, soy sauce was once considered exotic by most Westerners. They are a great resource for things like celeriac, fennel bulbs, salsify or other vegetables outside the realm of your typical supermarket.

They are also a good source for quality versions of the standards you still need which can't usually be gotten at a farmer's market: salt, butter, pasta, rice and the like. (Kudos to you if you're already among those who make their own butter, pasta or yogurt.) Maybe you'll just start with a red cabbage to make into a more fun version of your favorite coleslaw.

Or you might find that red and purple carrots with orange or yellow centers will renew the kids' interest in this common veggie. Be adventurous, even if it's not normally your nature- you're almost sure to discover something you love.

Annaprashana

Here's an idea to launch you on your way:

I propose a new holiday to commemorate the start of your new lifestyle. It is called "Annaprashana." It is the one day when you eat nothing for the entire day that isn't organic. Reminiscent of a Hindu ceremony (which was adapted from an earlier Buddhist tradition) celebrating a baby's first bite of solid food (which might also be called "real food"), we create a ceremony wherein we honor and memorialize our own first bites of "real food." As with the original event it is emblematic of the attempt to remove impurities from the body that were gotten in an earlier life.

The Hindu ceremony is typically held on the sixth day of the sixth month of the baby's life. Our holiday should be celebrated on June 6th, the sixth day of the sixth month of each year. In the traditional ceremony, a plate or plates are arranged containing objects which the baby is encouraged to touch— whatever she touches first is said to be auspicious sign as to the direction of her future life and career. In a similar vein at our holiday, for people with children in attendance or for those adults of a festive and whimsical nature, a temporary collage is created on a separate table or surface set aside for the purpose. Each participant brings one or more images or materials to the college which has meaning for them in relation to their relationship with food— a picture of a favorite food, a drawing of a scythe, leaves from a plant in the garden, a story telling the history of a favorite dish, a recipe, and photos of previous feasts with friends and family are all possibilities. Revive your storytelling skills. Everyone is encouraged to discuss the object they brought and its special meaning for them.

While great care is taken that all food eaten this day should be organic, the "focal" meal at which friends and family gather is composed of simple, unadorned foods emphasizing vegetables from the early Spring planting. However, it is important to have a universal and representative food for a holiday, I therefore declare asparagus to be the symbolic vegetable of our Annaprashana.

Like our new life, asparagus, when first started in the garden, needs some specific preparation and planning. It gets off to a slow start, as some of us may when attempting to transition to a completely organic diet. But once established, it flourishes year after year, bursting forth with vibrant energy in early Spring. It increases its yield as it ages, much as we will see an increased return on our investment in health as time goes on. Well tended, an asparagus patch can last for more than twenty years. It is a symbol of vigor and longevity, the quintessential icon for the life we're creating.

I can envision hunks of homemade bread with fresh farmer's cheese made from local goat milk, a chunky asparagus soup made with new potatoes, a sorrel salad and a crisp organic Ceago Sauvignon Blanc from California. On the other hand, a moment's search turned up a recipe online for fresh ricotta ravioli with snap peas, asparagus, and just-picked oregano, a perfect June dish. So, start your own family tradition. This is a joyous celebration of gratefulness and great hope for the future, reflecting a purification of the body and an expectation of renewed health and vitality. Happy Annaprashana! A votre santé.

Worry about your waste, not your waist

Now you've acquired the practice of purchasing good healthy food. So, what becomes of it? According to a recent study, more than 40% of all food produced in America is not eaten.[3] American families throw away an average of almost $600 worth of food per year, three times the amount tossed twenty years ago.[4] Nationwide household food waste alone adds up to $43 billion, making it a serious economic problem. Moreover, of that 30 million tons of wasted food, all but 2% winds up in landfills.[5] Rotting food in landfills creates methane as it decomposes and methane is a significant source of greenhouse gasses, which are implicated in global warming. Whew! What you do really does make a difference.

What to do about it all? Planning. Keep at least a mental note of the foods you have on hand, particularly perishables. Consider the meals that can be made from those foods and plan on having them over the next three or four days. One trick would be to resist the conventional Western approach to a meal, in which planning begins with the meat. We tend to think: "I'll have hamburgers," or "I'll make chicken," and everything else becomes a side dish. Start, instead with brown rice or pasta as the foundation and either plan to add a small amount of chicken, beef, fish or beans to the rice or pasta, or prepare something from them which will go on top.

When you start with brown rice, for instance, as your focal point, you can make extra, add completely different accessories the next night and have a completely different dish. Even better, try new grains; quinoa, buckwheat, millet are just a few of the nutrient-packed grains many folks haven't experienced yet.

Unlike 30 years ago, today these treats are readily available all over the country. Most of them cook quicker than rice and add a novel texture or slightly different taste to otherwise familiar dishes. Don't think you have to add sultanas and slivered almonds just because you're fixing millet, for instance. Try it with tomato sauce and dollops of ricotta. Go crazy. If experimenting isn't your thing yet, there are thousands of wonderful recipes on the Internet.

Consider stir-fries for dinner, or get creative and go with a soup or stew. (It doesn't have to be time consuming if made with leftovers. Keep some vegetable broth on hand.) Nothing says a hearty gnocchi/ chicken soup with root vegetables can't be served with buttered asparagus spears on the side. Or that brown rice with white fish and a spicy lemon yogurt sauce can't be served with a side of steamed collard greens drizzled with sautéed garlic and olive oil or a small side of pickled beets. This is your meal, make what you like.

You may need to pick up one or two items to complete a recipe, even if it's one you're inventing. Don't make the mistake of buying impulse items when you're there. Before you do go shopping, make that grocery list and take it with you so you don't forget the things you went for and wind up with a crazy array of seemingly disassociated foodstuffs (unless you're as adventurous as my sister!)

The recent changes in the world economy will probably be a benefit to the problem of growing landfills. Yes, our current troubles will have a positive side, though it may not seem like it. We should not long for the days of our callous extravagance but realize what careless fools we've been, with a renewed desire to change. We can seize this opportunity, this downsizing, to make wiser choices. Now is exactly the time to reshape our lives: to reconsider our approach to food, to free ourselves from relentless commitments on our time, and to rebuild bonds with those who matter to us most. I expect people will become more thoughtful about their choices, and more careful about their waste.

Remember, always, that you don't want your food to go bad. This is not the attitude we've had in recent decades. A past era in which, not wanting to *eat* bad food, one cavalierly tossed the food away if it appeared less than magazine-cover perfect, or if we'd simply forgotten precisely how long something may have been lingering on a shelf.

I'm talking about mentally tracking items in the fridge each time you open it and not allowing anything to become old, soft, brown, or inedible. Are the fresh lemons drying out? Maybe you should have that frozen fish tonight. Bananas going brown? Muffins in the morning. Make the batter the night before and stick it in the fridge.

The most important principle to hold close is the understanding that food is precious. Food is invaluable. Every member of the family should learn to do the "shelf scan" as they reach for milk or juice. What a great chance for children to learn to observe the changes in food and to take on the responsibility of a watchful assistant in the kitchen. (Even better if it can be used to jumpstart a conversation on anaerobic versus aerobic decomposition, or the aging process in the cycles of life.)

One more aspect of reducing waste is remembering to eat those leftovers. Did someone make a lasagna large enough for a family of eight, but there are only the four of you eating? Put half into the freezer. Have it a week later when you just don't feel like cooking. Leftover salad? Make soup. Yes, all those ingredients can go into a soup, even with vinaigrette already on it. I've done it. Just add a bit of this and that and you'll have something spectacular.

Leftover potatoes? Make potato bread or shepherd's pie. It's amazing how many people throw away food because they're unsure of how long it *might* last or just through laziness and failure to devote a small amount of attention to it. When the components of your meal actually become items of value, creativity begins to flow.

Here's another idea: *plan* to have leftovers. Maybe "Salmagundi Monday" can become a new tradition where every family member gets to choose the dish of their choice from the freezer that night, for reheating. (Just don't microwave it in the plastic freezer container.) Or maybe divvy up your leftovers and wrap them in foil for adult work lunches or kid lunches on the weekend. (Foil is a good choice because it will remind you not to microwave the plastic.)

Be aware of how you cook in terms, not only of your storage, but your cooking methods as well as utensils. This is all about your health and the health of future generations. In today's world, we must be mindful of the many ways in which our foods can be adulterated. Plastics, as we now know, exude breakdown chemicals like Bisphenol-A and other pseudo-estrogens when heated. It is possible that these chemicals are leached out even at room temperature when they are in contact with acids or oils or maybe any liquids.

These unnatural estrogens pervade the food we eat and have been implicated as playing a role in endocrine system cancers such as breast, ovarian and prostate cancers, in stunting the sexual maturation of young boys, and early puberty in girls, and in numerous neurological disorders, among other things.

The danger of chemicals defiling our foods comes, not only through how the food is raised— the pesticides, the fertilizers, the quality of the water, —but in how they are cooked and stored, by manufacturers as well as in our own homes. It is sometimes easy to overlook the contribution we, ourselves, are making in despoiling our foods when these activities have become as universal and commonplace as using Tupperware and oven roasting bags.

A few years back I was among those honored at a thank-you breakfast thrown by a group of volunteers in the sustainable food movement. We were to be served eggs. The concept behind the breakfast was lovely – the paid staff were being thanked by the volunteers for all their time and hard work.

At first, it seemed a unique way to assure that each got the omelet of their choice: every individual received a plastic bag and was instructed to write our name on it. Further down the line, there was a woman who scooped the already scrambled eggs from a large pot into our bags, then we were instructed to continue the line to the condiment counter where we could choose from already diced tomatoes, peppers, onion, shredded cheese, etc.

The bags were collected at the end of the line and I had expected that they would be dumped into a frying pan one after another, back in the kitchen. I envisioned several "chefs" keeping track as the omelets were cooked. I was shocked by what I saw. These eggs and their trappings were going to be boiled *in their plastic bags* and returned to us in the bag. I stepped out of the line holding my bag of eggs and peppers.

I tried quietly to get across, first to one host then another, that it was a really bad idea to cook any food in plastic, no less a form of plastic which was never intended to be boiled or even heated.

The organizer looked at me blankly, then got angry. She said, "We do this all the time at RV gatherings and it's fine. No one has ever gotten sick!" I was floored by the ignorance of such a statement by someone whose daily work involved teaching about organic agriculture and environmental health. I tried to explain that it would be a long term affect. I was met with a glare and urged aside. I chose to slip away to another nearby kitchen and heat my own egg in a cast iron skillet rather than "ruin" anyone else's breakfast.

Someday people will wonder why we ever did some of the things these last few generations have done to our food and our planet. This information is filtering slowly into the mainstream; my goal in writing this is that it reach the mainstream faster. It is important that we realize now. These are the kinds of things that build up in our systems and ruin, not breakfasts, but lives. How many more cancers will it take before we consider the long term effects of the things we ingest?

I advocate preventing any hot food from coming in contact with plastic, and except for the freezer, try to store things in glass or ceramic or foil. Sometimes, when an item is at risk of losing moisture, I will wrap it in paper or foil first, then put it in a re-purposed plastic grocery bag. When a product unavoidably arrives from its source in plastic, like a gallon of apple cider vinegar, I transfer it to a glass container for storage. I know that it's already been on the shelf for a while in its container, but I feel that I can perhaps prevent any *further* leaching. I simply try to do what I can, whenever I can. It's all we can do.

Another consideration: I always keep an inexpensive ceramic bowl and small plate and silverware with me at work, either in a locker, a drawer or tucked away somewhere, depending on the job. Nearly every company or work situation these days provides a microwave somewhere. It is not only safer, but a real plate and real flatware seems to make my meal more real, more noteworthy. It's another way of ascribing value to the food you are about to eat.

When truck driving I would sometimes just stop at a gas station or convenience store and bring my food inside in my own ceramic containers. (I'd usually also bring my ceramic mug and get a coffee and no one ever minded.) It's something to keep in mind if you travel.

A final note on the topic of not letting food go bad: a quick mention of expiration dates. I don't care much for expiration dates because I believe they usually reflect either a questionably fabricated shelf life or an excessively cautious "hurry up and buy more" implication by the manufacturer. But I am fortunate to be able to get goat milk from a neighbor and meat from my barn.

Kshamavaani

For those who don't have that luxury, this note: many people don't seem to realize that the expiration date refers to the product BEFORE it is opened. If it's November 10th and the yogurt stamp says it's good until December 16th, that means "only if you haven't opened it." Once you've opened it and exposed it to air, all bets are off and it will decompose within its usual time. (Three to four days for some things, a week or so for others, like yogurt. That's why people can't believe the milk has gone bad when the expiration date is a week later. If you opened it, it won't last. It may take a little adjustment, but it's really no big deal to regularly glance over the shelves in the fridge and formulate your battle plan.

Eyes Bigger Than Your Stomach

Another facet of reducing waste, as well as reducing your waist, is to know how much a portion is.

Americans love to get a deal. A yard sale, a flea market, the lottery, the stock market, we all dream of getting something for nothing. That mindset extends to our eating habits. The marketing of this "something for nothing" notion is one small part of the overarching machine that exists to get you to eat more than you your body wants, to buy more than you need.

So when it comes to eating out, people have become accustomed to seeing large portions. People expect large portions. People demand large portions, or they feel cheated. In all but the most upscale restaurants, and even in many of them over the last two decades, portion sizes have gotten larger. I once overheard a conversation between a group of acquaintances who dined out together at various mid-range restaurants once a week. When asked if the food at the place she had recommended was any good, one woman said by means of endorsement: "No, it's not great, but the portions are huge!" *What??!*

Much of the marketing for this mindset is aimed directly and blatantly at men. The "man-sized" meal, "eating like a man" are common advertising tactics making reference to mountains of (usually) greasy, bland junk food. Young men especially fall easily to this enticement, and in my observation, are often prone to fill up competitively, as a way of proving that they are now men. Middle aged and older men often do the same as a way of proving that they are still young. I suspect that in groups of men eating together, each will eat more than any one of them would eat if alone.

As an example there is actually a television show on the Travel Channel called *Man vs. Food*. The overweight host travels from city to city throughout the US seeking the largest, greasiest meals he can find. He consumes them on air in a kind of spectacle of gleeful debauchery. The episode I saw had him sitting down to a 7+ lb. burger with mushrooms, cheese & onions –described by the restaurant's owner as enough to feed eight people– and trying to down the whole thing in less than an hour.

Let it be noted that dieticians currently suggest 3 oz of meat is an appropriate portion for a meal for an adult. That would make this burger, containing 4 lbs of meat, large enough, in fact, to feed *twenty-one* people. This fool made himself feel sick in the process of attempting to wolf down a seven pound burger. He gave up partway through, and wasted the rest of the food on his plate, including a mandatory side of fries which were not even touched. This, in a city where, like all cities, people undoubtedly went to bed hungry that night.

Women fall prey in a more subtle way to this facet of marketing as evidenced by the woman's comments above, but they are less overtly targeted in this regard. However they, too, take the bait of seeing a larger plate as something needing to be filled. In America, it seems, better a whole mountain of mediocre food than tiny portions of exquisite cuisine.

In our faux-classless, jeans-wearing, cowboy-fetishist society, the media would have us believe that only fey tubercular poets eat "cuisine." A real man has worked up a roaring appetite roping cattle since dawn or felling trees. A real man could eat a horse. With ketchup. The problem is that most men today actually sit behind a desk, stand behind a counter, or use machinery and automation to remove any break-a-sweat labor from their work. Women typically expend even less energy moving through their daily tasks, for a variety of reasons. Yet, in the American self-image, proffered and fomented by savvy advertisers, we see ourselves as dynamic, rugged pioneers in Big Country, with Big Dreams and Big Appetites. The sad truth is, the only thing *big* is us.

It takes maturity to recognize that we are being manipulated. It takes a level of self-reflection and courage to say "You know what? I'm not going to be one of the pack"; to realize that the calories you burn in a day are far fewer than some product pusher wants you to believe. It takes a self-assured man to order the junior burger, knowing that it will be enough to fill him up.

Begin to see mountains of greasy, doughy "feed" as beneath you. Stand up to the ad execs who are so convinced they can make you cave through some form of peer pressure. Order the smaller sizes. Better yet, bring food from home; save that ten dollars a day spent on lunch and buy better geek gear. Find a place to eat outdoors. Or eat at your desk or breakroom and then go for a walk. You never know what you might find.

Once you obtain a modicum of distance from the infernal noise of the marketing machine, you begin to see portion sizes big enough to choke a hippo as an insult. What do they think you look like? A baleen whale ready to suck in everything around you? Send your food back. Sure, not eating all of it is theoretically an option, but study after study has shown that we are a people who dutifully attempt to clean our plates. We all know that it's much harder to decide when we're done if there's still food on the plate.

Satiety, the feeling of fullness and satisfaction we seek when eating, is a matter of signals sent from the stomach to the brain. It has been established that these signals take 20 minutes or so to reach the brain from the time we begin eating. If you've snarfed everything on your plate in ten minutes, your "stomach" (actually your brain) doesn't even know you've eaten yet!

In our culture this usually means that we will continue eating until nearly all the food around us is gone. This is a bad choice. It's what makes us pile on the pounds and feel bloated, overfull and guilty later. Eating more slowly is clearly a better way to eat.

For now, we want restaurants to know we won't accept mounds of dull, second-rate fare. Even if food is regularly left behind, we are not sending the message that the portion is too large back to the cook in the kitchen by leaving part of it on our plate— it's a busboy or waitron who glumly removes the trash from the tables. So we're sending it back to the cook. Let the kitchen know that you take exception to being seen as a human dispose-all and you would like half of the food (or a particular food item) removed from your plate. Reclaim your dignity.

Portion extortion
(A little something extra...)

As much as we waste, we are still consuming nearly 50% more than in decades past, often almost unwittingly. At the National Heart, Lung and Blood Institute website,[7] research shows that single portions of many common lunch and dinner items eaten outside the home have grown exponentially in just the last 20 years. A few examples:

	20 Years Ago	Today	Increase
One cheeseburger	333 calories	590 calories	**257 *extra* calories**
One portion of spaghetti and meatballs	500 calories (1c. pasta/ sauce, 3 meatballs)	1,025 calories (this includes **2** c. pasta/ sauce and 3 gigantic meatballs)	**525 *extra* calories**
One portion of French fries	210 calories (typically 2.4 oz.)	610 calories (today's portion averages 6.9 oz.)	**400 *extra* calories**
A turkey sandwich	320 calories	820 calories (usually nearly 10" long)	**500 *extra* calories**
One chocolate chip cookie	55 calories (1 ½" dia.)	275 calories (usually 5" in dia.)	**220 *extra* calories**

Kshamavaani

You may think, "I only had a turkey sub, a soda and a cookie for lunch, it's really not that much."

The real deal though, is that while you may have had the "same" lunch as someone 20 years ago, you've just eaten, in a single meal, 885 *more* calories than the meal would have provided back then. If you are a woman of average height, and fairly sedentary activity level, this would be *three quarters* of your needed calories for the entire day.[8] [One turkey sub (820 cal), chocolate chip cookie (275 cal), 20 oz soda (250 cal) total: 1345 calories.] So, even when you try to cut back to a reasonable few items, it's nearly impossible to purchase a meal of moderate proportions. Yet another reason to make your own lunch.

Even drinks— *especially* drinks, are important to consider when assessing your food-health lifestyle. Did you know that Coca-cola's famous contoured soda bottle contained 6.5 oz for almost the first 40 years of its existence?

Yet in 2006, a *medium* fountain soda at McDonald's or Burger King was 21 oz., a large was 32 oz. and an even bigger 42 oz. size was sold at many fast food places. The 42 oz. soda is 410 calories by itself. Even if you are an active male, that one drink is nearly ¼ of your entire daily requirement of calories.

I don't recommend counting calories at every meal. It is not a desirable way to live. It focuses on the wrong aspects of the food in front of you. That food is a treasure, a gift. It should be something anticipated and then savored slowly like a book that's so good you don't want it to end. If your food doesn't impart this message to you, take a closer look at your what you're eating and reconsider your choices. Eat better quality food.

As for calories, a vague sense of calorie requirements is all that is necessary. Know this: the average person needs roughly 2000 calories a day. Use this as a reference. It's good enough to have a broad, loose sense that:

a) *About* 1800 calories are what you might need in a day if you are a woman, *about* 2200 if you are a man.

And,

b) Too many calories are bad.

Keep these two thoughts in mind, then take a glance at the calorie count of your items if you enter a fast food place. If a quick tally of your average meal runs 1000 or above, that lunch is more than you should have for half the day. Or think of it this way: no one meal should be more than 600-700 calories. If you drink two 20 oz. sodas a day, that is one quarter of your entire day's worth of allotted calories.

Soon you can make the leap to realizing that if a typical portion of spaghetti and meatballs runs 1,025 calories, (more than half a day's worth) then a mountain of fried chicken strips with hush puppies and fries is *also* going to be more than you need, whether or not you have a nutrition label or a calculator nearby.

If a turkey sub is already 820 calories, you don't need to read a warning to know that an equal-sized triple cheese and three-meat sub will be far, far more than you need at one meal.

In fact, the act of eating out can begin to seem like a dangerous and ridiculous activity. An organization called the Centre for Science in the Public Interest, an advocacy group, recently studied the steakhouse favorite: cheese fries with ranch dressing. It contains about 3,000 calories, way more than the *total* recommended daily calories for an active adult male. And it's a side dish. Worse, this dish alone contained 11 grams of trans fat and 81 grams of saturated fat. Is it any wonder we're overweight?

A good guide to help you understand portion sizes is to remember the amount in a visual way. A classic example is this guideline [9]—

An appropriate serving of vegetables or fruit is about the size of your fist.

A serving of pasta is about the size of one scoop of ice cream. (Less than the size of your fist.)

A serving of meat, fish, or poultry is the size of a deck of cards or the size of your palm (minus the fingers).

A serving of snacks such as chips should be no more than about the size of a cupped handful.

A serving of apple is the size of a baseball. (Hmmm. About the size of your fist.)

A serving of potato is the size of a computer mouse. (Not any bigger than your fist.)

A serving of bagel is the size of your palm.

A serving of pancake is the size of a compact disc. (Use a gravy ladle as a dipper.)

A serving of steamed rice is the size of a cupcake wrapper. (About ½ the size of your fist.)

A serving of cheese is the size of your whole thumb (from the tip to the base).

But lets make it even easier. If you read through the list, you see that no single portion of anything should be larger than your fist. Many dense items like meat and cheese should be smaller. There you go, there's a reference that is always "handy."

If this seems like a shockingly small amount, it is because we have become accustomed to eating gargantuan, obscene amounts of food. It's time now to seek out not quantity, but quality. When we crave "lots, lots, lots" we are expressing another facet of the "Endless Child." Not only do we want immediate gratification, we want more than we need, more than we even feel hungry for, we want it all just because it is there.

I believe that soon the time will come when this kind of expression of gluttony will be seen as an embarrassment. Our social norms will change back to the way they were through most of human history, when people gorging themselves to the point of queasiness were seen, rightfully, as pigs. Our middle class have been eating like poor folk who've never been invited to the table before—we pile our plate high, we grab the largest portions, we go back for thirds. Composure, coolness and mature detached restraint have fled the dining room.

But once one reacquires those abilities, it is even possible to feel an uncomfortable aversion to acquaintances who act with such abased self-indulgence. This isn't to say that we should harken back to the days of Victorian England where all was pomp and façade, not at all. There is room somewhere between loutish behavior and pretense, for simple self-control.

Early generations of Americans knew the self-conscious disquiet of being seen as a swinish boor. That attitude has since been renounced by advertisers for whom *more* and *bigger* are the only path to profit. Nearly all other cultures still have a strong sense of genteel mortification at American-sized portions.

I remember many years ago, my Japanese roommate in NYC trying to teach me to make nori-maki. With bashful but irrepressible giggling she tried to explain that the size of my amateur roll and its resultant slices was considered crass and indelicate. It was rude.

Thoroughly a product of the bigger-is-always-better American mindset, I struggled to understand. My slices were the size I'd seen in American markets. I learned for the first time that American portions were seen in much of the rest of the world as graceless and unseemly: gauche.

We need to overcome the sense of feeling cheated when we see smaller portions on our plate. To do this, we need to learn to court quality. First we must reacquire the expectation of excellence in the foods we consume. By this I refer back to the mindset of not seeing our meals as something trifling to fill us up in the moment.

When the food before us becomes, not just a snootful of mush to chow down on, but actually the embodiment of our future health, it gains value. That meal has a purpose. Its purpose is to wean us off our medications. Its purpose is to enable us to jump for joy. This is the promise of real food. When you can look at tomatoes or broccoli or snowpeas and anticipate not just a crisp succulent burst of garden-fresh flavor but your own vigor and potentiality, you have begun to see food for what it really is.

We have become accustomed to thinking of our food in terms of our weight and the calories provided. In this way of thinking, foods are interchangeable. If I want to eat ice cream at lunch I might skip the toast and omelet at breakfast and my calorie count will be roughly the same. I am passing up potentially quality foods for less nutrition, but still "keeping to my diet."

This is only one reason why this is not a good approach to eating. Instead of calories, we must learn to start thinking in terms of its life energy. Obviously these are not an assessment of the same property. A calorie is a measurement of the potential heat to be expended by something one eats, but that is not what calorie counters are considering when weighing and counting. At some level, ultimately, they are thinking "how is this food product going to affect the way I look?"

The purpose of seeing food as life energy is to get away from thinking of foods in terms of how they make us look ("if I eat this cheesecake it will make me fat, if I eat this celery it will make me thin,") and begin to think about how much a food item is contributing to our health.

Now, those folks who are analytically inclined, who need numbers and Brix measurements and calorie counters, scales, gadgets and the like, may find it difficult to accept the concept of life energy. It is not something that can be tallied in the lab, nor something determined by thermometers, hygrometers, Geiger counters, mass spectrometers or even some fancy Chromo Tomographic Hyperspectral Imaging Sensor.

No, it's more a measure of a kind of common sense. It's something that the average person can understand with the merest whisper of effort and attention. It is a metaphorical assessment of how far removed from its original purpose (to us) a particular plant or animal might be, as we prepare to eat it. It might help to think, when reaching for a product, "How far has this apple fallen from the tree?"

In the elements of each dish, each food product has a certain amount of life energy to give to us depending on what it has gone through to get to our plate. Raw foods, as any raw food proponent will tell you, contain the most life energy. Think about it—those plants are not making the food for us, they are storing or producing food for the continued life of their species, and they pour all their energy into the process.

Seeds and sprouts, especially, are bursting with all the life energy that plant will need to form itself into a whole plant. Peas and beans are seeds, as are whole uncut grains, containing the "germ" of the future generation. Eggs, by the same measure, are full of life energy.

Roots and leaves are the places for storage or processing. They are the plant's warehouses, and are, at the right time of year, stocked with life energy. Stems, on the other hand, are usually just the highway-not bad for you but not really of great value in terms of life energy, which is why we don't eat a lot of stems. In plant foods, not all that food energy is available to us to digest and, at times, processes like cooking, fermentation, or soaking with lime can help our species to assimilate its nutrients. One step removed from the tree is sometimes beneficial.

Meats have a lot of life energy, they are the muscles where the animal stores its energy or the organs on which the continued vitality of that animal depends. Skin is not a source of life energy, although it comes from an animal; it's not a source of power for the animal or a storage place for energy. That's why we rarely eat the skins of animals. Fruits are a tidy package of the food the seeds will need to thrive so they contain a lot of quick energy but without the depth of life energy that the seed itself will have (for the plant. Obviously not all seeds and pits are edible.)

Fruit is excellent for you, but as a dessert, a treat. Honey is in a similar category. As nectar produced by the plants to entice pollination by insects, it's food for the bees and other pollinators, it is not the life entity itself. It contains a lot of micronutrients and as such is far better for health than white sugar, but honey should be considered a treat.

Fats and oils, when fresh and cold-pressed, or in the case of butters, churned up from milk, are full of life energy. This is where a plant or animal keeps its stores, to be converted to energy when needed.

This is why it is so important to choose organic fats and oils, because your body will be holding onto these components for the long term, as well as all the fat-soluble toxins which cling to them.

White sugar goes through considerable processing before it arrives on our plate, any micronutrient value the sap of the cane may have had for the plant remains in the molasses. White sugar, like white flour, is completely devoid of any life energy by the time it reaches you, as is anything that has been powdered, dried, refined and reconstituted. Each step of processing leaves a part of the original product's life energy behind.

With some plants, as mentioned, little of the plant's benefit would have been available to us without some form of processing, so although life energy is lost, we still gain something from a single level of removal from its original state. But with each successive rung of processing, more life energy is lost until, at times, there is virtually nothing there.

Among these levels of processing we have to include not just active steps like milling, cooking, drying, freezing, freeze-drying, and reconstituting, but storage. Each time the product sits, exposed to the air, its life force dissipates out of it. Understand that this is different than what is meant by shelf life.

When manufacturers attempt to extend shelf life, they are usually trying to prevent actual spoilage, that is, the enjoyment of that product by organisms other than ourselves, most often bacteria. In general the approach they take is to strip the product of as much of its life force as is feasible while still maintaining its look and some semblance of its taste. This is done through the use of things like chemical adulterants, multi-faceted processing steps or irradiation.

At this point, as noted earlier, even the bacteria are reluctant to partake of the result. Now we can begin to understand why decoy foods are so bad for us, even without the pesticides, sewage sludge and what-all that went into growing the original ingredients. Each step in the processing of a natural product saps it. A piece of chicken breast that has been decomposed into a slush, heated, cooled, dissolved, diluted, filled with synthetic flavor enhancers and stabilizers, reformulated into a shapeless glob, and then cooked in plastic wrap which leaches chemicals into its molten form has actually become an anti-life energy product.

What we are aiming for instead is to make use of that nutritious nugget before its life energy is dispersed or depleted. We want to consume it as early as possible after harvest, be it animal or vegetable, and in as unprocessed a state as possible. This is clearly another advantage to eating locally grown foods.

However, some amount of preservation and processing are inevitable, everything cannot always be consumed in the moment, and some methods are even desirable. Freezing is a way of preserving, not all, but most of the substance's life energy. Cooking often makes vegetable nutrients available which otherwise wouldn't be, and increases the safety of eating meats. Another ancient and valuable method of preserving food, while often also increasing its benefit to us, is fermentation.

The recent resurgence in popularity of vegetable fermentation in the West is due not only to the increased digestibility of the finished product, but the added enzymes and antibiotic substances created by the beneficial bacteria. "We are finding that fermented cabbage could be healthier than raw or cooked cabbage, especially for fighting cancer," says Finland researcher Eeva-Liisa Ryhanen, Ph.D.[10] Cabbage is only one of the many vegetables commonly fermented. On every inhabited continent there have been traditional fermented foods.[11]

Though maybe we can't measure it, once we begin to think of food in terms of life energy we understand why a product made of white flour, white sugar, hydrogenated fats and synthetic flavorings has nothing to offer us. Synthetic or refined nutrient "enhancement" of these products is nothing more than a new outfit for the emperor. The only real food is not far removed from the garden.

Smaller portions of really quality foods, then, will provide us with the same (or better) nutrient levels as mammoth portions of refined processed foods, and with fewer calories. The problem becomes convincing ourselves that we've had enough when our eyes are accustomed to expecting more.

What will help us choose to eat less is to relearn the act of tasting. The simple act of eating slowly, of prying out the flavors and taking notice of the combinations of spice or texture will help us to more fully enjoy these gifts of nourishment. It will also help us to feel full while having eaten less.

Remember, your stomach doesn't register a feeling of satiety until 20 minutes or so after you've begun eating. That's why the food may be gone but you're still hungry. You grab seconds, or maybe some more rolls and butter. You eat the food you were going to save for later in the week. Then, 10-15 minutes later you feel ill.

By eating more slowly your stomach will catch up with your plate. To start, we must begin to think of our meals in terms of small amounts of delightful tastes worthy of notice. It will pay to bear in mind this comment, made by a visiting French chef way back in 1893:

> "I cannot protest enough against the custom so general in the United States to give to the table only the necessary time and to eat like a locomotive taking water, by doing which you expose yourself to the various stomach diseases which make so rapidly the fortune of the doctors and druggists."[12]

"Everyone eats and drinks, but few appreciate taste."
~ Confucius (551-479 BC)

Although there are those who would argue that the superior flavor of fresh organic vegetables, fruits and meats is clearly evident when compared to conventional food, this may not seem the case to you if you haven't yet fully learned to taste.

In the womb, our species has the biological potential to accept almost limitless taste preferences, from curry to crickets to caribou to cola and everything in between. Yet even in this early state, our propensity is beginning to be influenced by what our mother eats as we develop. And there's the rub.

The better part of several generations of Americans have been acclimated from earliest development to the bland, high sugar, high salt Western diet. From birth on, the majority of people in Western society then consume foods with extraordinary levels of added sweeteners.

[Did you know that when Oreo cookies were first introduced in China, people wouldn't eat them. They had to be reformulated to be less sweet in order to be palatable to the Chinese, who haven't yet developed our sugar addiction.][13]

It often isn't possible to simply "start liking other foods" if you're someone who hasn't done much experimenting. The process has to be conscious and an effort will have to be made, but the rewards are great.

Begin with observation. Most of us eat familiar foods with scant regard for visual presentation. In a restaurant, an obligatory sprig of parsley is pushed to the side as we dive in. When we went to a fast food joint, all of our attention was drawn to the wrapper's glitzy colors- we often didn't even remove it, just peeled it back before grabbing a bite. Now we are going to contemplate the things we eat.

If your food isn't worth a few moments of appreciative reflection, is it really worth eating? Below, for fun, is an idea for a new approach to a dinner shared with friends, based on the elements of a classic wine tasting.

~The Wine Tasters Guide To Food Tasting~

Everyone is gathered and seated. Food is brought to the table.

1 - *Appearance*

Each diner is encouraged to look at the colors, the confluence of items displayed, the interplay of shapes. Share with each other your delight in the details, either intentional or accidental: tiny shards of lemon peel against a dark green leaf, the beautiful golden curl of a puff pastry, the dance of pine nuts encircling a bowl of Brussels sprouts and cranberries.

You do not have to carve your watermelon into a swan or arrange your chives into Chinese characters to create visual marvels in a meal. They're already there. Enjoy the gentle undulations of a single green bean. And take the time to look around the room, feel the pleasure of the setting, the company.

As the food is being served you might want to think of a word or phrase that would describe the meal's presentation. Is it playful? Bold and flamboyant? Darkly exotic? A modern monochrome? The picture of elegant austerity? Or maybe you want to come up with the names for all the different colors of green in the salad or vegetable dish.

Make each other laugh. Describe the color palette of the entrée in as many ways as you can. A breaded, broiled fish might be ivory with soft washes of silver, glistening in delicate pools of warm sunshine, flecked with the amber, sienna, saffron and goldenrod of bread crumbs, and stippled with ruby specks of cayenne.

Be lavish and luxurious in your descriptions. Enchant one another. Awaken in yourselves the visual component of food. Learn to notice.

2 - The "Nose" or "Bouquet"

Take the time to inhale the aromas of a warm dish after it is brought to the table. Let it linger for a precious moment, savor the subtle fragrances. See what you can tell about the spices or ingredients of a dish before you've tasted it. What does it remind you of? What memories does it hold? The bouquet of a favorite dish can conjure some of life's most exquisite remembrances. Think about what you are sensing. Can you hold onto this aroma for the future?

3 - The "Mouth"

Finally, taste a small portion of something. Relish the textures, the interplay of sensations: tang, sweetness, sourness, tartness, bitterness, saltiness, astringency, finish. Find the umami, the fifth taste sense. (Umami is a meaty "fullness" of taste, not exclusive to meat, but found in things like real soy sauce as well. Its name means "yummy" in Japanese. So there you go, find the yummy!)[14]

Try to sort out and name, if even to yourself, several distinct perceptions. Different elements of taste are perceived in different parts of the mouth, move a tiny bite of food around and notice differences in taste as you do. Does this culinary creation deliver on the promise of its bouquet? How does temperature play a role in the dish? Does a sauce caress its entrée or transfuse its ingredients? Do you prefer the texture of the crispy edges at the top of the casserole or the creamy warmth of the center? Does the fire of a hot curry sparkle across your tongue? Does the sharp sour of sorrel jab your salivary glands?

Follow with a small bite of a different dish and enjoy the parrying between sensations. Eating slowly comes naturally because you are finding your way through the meal as if for the first time. This is the kind of dinner party which can be had with familiar foods critiqued anew or with a meal based around the theme of a foreign culture or unaccustomed fare. Still, I suggest always having one dish which is something most people haven't tried before.

Now although it is more fun to share in the discovery of food with adventurous friends, learning to taste and bringing something novel to mealtime is something that can certainly be done alone or with family. Often years ago, when I found myself eating alone for a day, I would come up with themes and ideas to make my meals more fun. There is an element of this in the challenge of eating foods from entirely within a one hundred mile radius. Another angle is a meal which you have grown yourself, or have worked to acquire every element directly from nature, as Michael Pollen did in *Omnivore's Dilemma*.

I also did things like picking a letter of the alphabet and having every food have to start with that letter—this can be quite flexible and silly, of course: borscht with burgers and buns, fricasseed fish, fennel and focaccia, cheesy chorizo casserole, sautéed shrimp, shallots and summer squash on spaghetti, pasta with porcini-parmesan pomodoro. To the daily exercise of deciding what to eat, it can bring some lighthearted humor. This is something kids would enjoy. It's not cheating to look up recipe names online or to use a less common usage or the name of a vegetable in another language, eggplant becoming aubergine for example. That could very well be part of the fun (don't tell them they're learning.)

I began cooking at a very young age and quickly learned to feel confident around food— what a great assignment for a ten or eleven year old, (or older) —set aside one night a week where they can plan and execute a meal, with decreasing levels of supervision. The challenge of a single letter to work with could add an appealing element of child-age kookiness.

Another way to enjoy the diversity of gustatory sensations Mother Nature has to offer is by having a "taste test." I recently gathered three kinds of persimmons to determine which one I liked the best. The Hachiya and the Fuyu were from the co-op, and the small local one from a neighbor's yard. I chose all three based on their relatively equivalent firmness, placed them in a brown paper bag together, and waited expectantly until they were all equally ripe. When the time was right, I tried a slice of each one, slowly appraising its nuances. [I can't tell you which is best, you'll have to decide for yourself!]

This game can really open your eyes. Most middle aged and older folks know that commercial tomatoes have no taste, it has become a cliché. But maybe you've only heard that tomatoes are supposed to be great tasting; you don't know what the fuss is about –they don't taste that great to you. If you are a young person, under 30, then it is possible that you have never had the real, untainted version of the food that shares its name with what you are eating.

If you have lived on conventional fare and you've only had sliced tomatoes from fast food joints or in a prepackaged pseudo-salad, maybe you are not aware that a tomato really has a distinct and incredible flavor. Different varieties have different flavors. I highly recommend that you try the taste test with one or two never-refrigerated heirloom tomatoes from your local farmer's market and any common supermarket tomato. *(You do know that you should not refrigerate a tomato, right? It becomes mealy and loses flavor.)*

If you approach each sample with an earnest, "wine-taster's" evaluation, not only will you be stunned at the difference, you may begin to wonder why you've been deprived of real food throughout your life. Who are these people who have an economic incentive in creating the belief that what they offer is all that exists? How dare they?

When it comes to tastes, I like my food with a little zing, a little crunch. I like food that bites back. A hearty course bread, crisp vegetables, dishes with spice and flavor, around the world these are the tastes that nearly every nationality has cultivated. Babies are fed milder, sweeter fare while adults favor stronger, hotter, bitter, pungent flavors, from Polynesia to the Arctic.

If vibrant flavors are new to you, start slowly. Try a small amount of a dish, or make a spicy recipe at home using only half the amount of strong spices. Remember that, as a child, most of us probably didn't appreciate our first taste of wine or coffee.

The important issue is to broaden your horizons. At every evening meal, try to include a new taste. Sour or bitter or astringent vegetables are a good category for Americans to introduce to the menu. These vegetables are usually particularly high in vitamins; things like sorrel, dandelion, sauerkraut, or kimchi. Or try adding a few shreds of grated ginger to carrots, parsnips or fish. Add some mandarin orange or tangerine slices to a salad or stir-fry.

In no time you will find pleasure in the sweet tartness of a kiwi that makes your tongue curl up at the edges, or a zesty capsicum that clears your sinuses and opens your eyes. You'll learn to love the subtle lemongrass in a spicy Thai soup, the caraway seeds in a dark rye bread, the light tang of a fresh goat cheese.

At each meal, whether alone or in company, time should be spent noticing and preparing to enjoy what you are about to eat. Before you eat, as you pick up your fork, take a breath. Exhale. Now, take another longer, deeper breath. Exhale slowly. Relax. *Now* eat. From now on do this before putting anything in your mouth. Learn to take a quiet pride in the knowledge that the food you are eating and serving your family is of the highest quality.

Appreciation doesn't have to be only about taste or smell or color. Mull over what you know about each element as you prepare the food or as you are about to eat it. Think about how it was grown and preserved and how it got to you. Contemplate what you know of its value to your health. Does this food contain vitamin C? Is it something you're eating because of its useful fiber content? Are these greens you raised from seed?

Visualize the strength you are receiving. Be conscious of its life. All food was alive at one time, or should have been. If aspects of the food you had been eating were never part of the life of this planet, were made from molecules synthesized in a laboratory, could they really have been providing for your body at a cellular level?

Your new food, on the other hand, is to your cells as the perfect key is to a lock. You are unlocking captured sunshine with which to power your body.

Vandana Shiva tells us that in Indian culture a small prayer is often given to a garden plant:

"In you I will assume the cosmos resides and I will pay you reverence."

I believe the same to be true when that vegetable arrives on your plate. It carries within it the Essence, the All, and it can reside within you as long as you choose to continue the cycle. Revere it.

I envision an America where vast platters of insipid grub are not the norm; where even truckers prefer hunks of wholegrain bread served with thick, rustic, flavorful stews to plates of sodden macaroni mixed with squeeze-cheese food product. An America where pre-formed, plastic-encased meat slabs, distinguishable as ham or turkey only by salt level, will become a thing of the past.

Especially in these financially difficult times, food will gain esteem. People will become more demanding in their tastes, desiring not economic value, but excellence of their meals as we realize that health is a direct result of our connection to earth.

It can be achieved by our commitment to maintaining as short a link as possible between the soil and our daily sustenance. Medications are the anomaly. This recognition has already taken root.

Likewise, smaller portions will become the norm as it will once again be seen as gluttony to gorge one's self. It will be unnecessary to engage in such displays when our foods provide ample nutrients. Already people are choosing new dinnerware sets which offer smaller sized plates and bowls.

Cravings will stop when our cell's needs have been met. Disdain for hoarding and "hogging" will arise; these behaviors will be considered beneath the dignity of anyone who hasn't recently been rescued from 30 days in a dingy at sea. This day is surely coming.

May the circle be unbroken

Nevertheless, try as we might to reduce our waste by thoughtful planning, judicious portions, and creative re-purposing, we will have foods at home that have unavoidably gone bad. Scraps or peels, pits, coffee grounds or tea leaves, the outer leaves and stalks of things are inescapable waste. Or, maybe there will be an occasion when you don't have enough left on your restaurant plate to make a meal but you don't want it to go into the landfill. Good for you, for taking it home. But what to do with it?

Compost it. Take it home, bring it out into the yard and feed the earth. Composting is different from a landfill in that the food is not sitting on old plastic bags or sheets of drywall or whatever, but able to naturally decompose. Yes, this book is about food, but real food is dependant on the soil, which is created from vegetation. It's all part of the same cycle.

Kshamavaani

What you do with your garbage may one day have a direct effect on the quality of your comestibles –and sooner rather than later, if you use your compost on your garden. So let's talk for a moment about the miracle of reincarnation.

My compost pile is a 4' diameter of welded wire around five metal posts. That's all. No fancy expensive plastic rotating thing. Nothing to care for or tend. It does not attract flies or varmints, it does not smell. I simply dump the days vegetable scraps into the "pile" and in the summer when there's a risk of flies, throw a layer of lawn clippings or raked leaves on top. The welded wire or even chicken wire prevents the chickens as well as the raccoons, possums, coyotes and whatever else from getting into the pile.

And no, I don't rake leaves –I feel content to leave them where the trees drop them— but they are available for free from my county recycling center in bags brought in by others who do all the work for me. Your town may have a similar arrangement. Or maybe you can get bagged leaves from neighbors. In a previous city in which I lived, I would collect my neighbors bagged leaves from the curb before the city workers got to them.

Anything from nature can go into your compost pile, including animal parts. Nonetheless, you may want to avoid fats, bones, milk, and other animal products because they would be more likely to attract the attention of wild animals or your own pets, and because they don't decompose as quickly as vegetables. There are books and websites out there making composting sound as complicated and scientific as building a rocketship. Don't worry about it.

It certainly can be as complicated as you would like; you can buy thermometers, biological starters, rolling bins, strainers. You can buy aerators and keep charts; measure carbon vs. nitrogen; weigh browns and greens, whatever. But you don't have to. Maybe you just want to return your waste to the earth. Put it in a pile. Cover it with leaves. Every two years or so, move the fencing a few feet to the side and start a new pile. That's it.

If you actually want to use the resultant magnificent fertile soil on your garden, you will have to refrain from putting pet feces in the pile and possibly from including weed seeds as well.

You may want to investigate composting further and speed up your de-comp with tools and bacteria, watering and turning. But the point is that it isn't necessary if you don't intend to *use* the compost and yet, you have still contributed back to the earth.

That 4' to 5' diameter of earth is richer for the offering you've given. While it may not seem like much (especially because you're not wasting as much as you used to,) imagine millions of people doing the same all over the country. And every year or two moving to a new spot. Over time it becomes quite a substantial bit of ground. It also means that inedible vegetable matter isn't festering inside plastic bags at a dump. It means it didn't have to be trucked somewhere. You can think of the earth as your giant pet, and that little fenced circle, its mouth. You feed it with each day's scraps. And those scraps are turned back into a beautiful soil: earth.

Even in the densest asphalt jungles, you may not have a tiny plot of earth to call your own but there is surely a spot of soil somewhere. Do a little inquiring about the neighborhood. Most cities in the US today, as well as other parts of the world, have vibrant, active community gardens whose members might be delighted to accept your strictly vegetable compostables.

Or consider getting into vermicomposting- the increasingly popular practice of using earthworms to turn vegetable scraps into an incredibly rich potting soil additive called castings. This can be done in an even smaller area than a compost pile—under the sink in a box. It is easy to discreetly deposit worm castings in a local patch of weeds on your way to work. Throw in a few flower seeds and create your own secret little neighborhood garden. If your life is so unfortunately urban that you never encounter the outdoors, but go from parking garage to parking garage, get some houseplants. Worm castings are a wonderful medium for windowsill gardening.

Kshamavaani

Whatever you do, do something. And remember that Kshamavaani represents forgiveness. This is not the time for blaming yourself for past waste or ostentation. Don't worry about last year, or yesterday or this morning. Every single moment throughout each day is your starting point. It is a movement of passive resistance, but it is also an internal movement, inside you. Work with the 90/10 rule. It allows the flexibility to make choices. The only real act is to energize your resolve in the choice of organic, simple eating and to persevere in that decision with a confident vision of a better future.

Always choose from the position of being an adult, of using what you know in your heart, above all, being honest with yourself. Results will not have the immediacy that a two-year old would be satisfied with, we are working for the long term. In the words of an old Chinese proverb: "One generation plants the trees; another gets the shade." As grownups, we can handle that. It can be a source of healthy pride to give to the future.

Steel yourself to distractions; there will be those who will try to undermine you. For instance, expect huge distressing propaganda campaigns promoting the safety of irradiated foods; cloned foods and nanotechnology. Follow the money and you'll see what's really behind the huckstering. Stand firm. You are not alone, but without you it will not work. This is a movement which will change the direction of our culture. The act of Kshamavaani is also considered the first step in the path to liberation. This is your path, your liberation.

CHAPTER 7

Into the Freylakh*

(*also the name of a great Klezmer band)

"There can never be good for the bee which is bad for the hive."
~ Ralph Waldo Emerson

"We cannot live for ourselves alone.
Our lives are connected by a thousand invisible threads,
and along these sympathetic fibers, our actions run as
causes and return to us as results."
~ Herman Melville

John F. Kennedy said "Peace is a daily, a weekly, a monthly process, gradually changing opinions, slowly eroding old barriers, quietly building new structures." I would say that the same goes for any type of change we commit to making in the world.

Learning to view our sustenance as valuable will not come easily after nearly 50 or 60 years of being trained otherwise. True, it is the only thing you really need to do. But there are other endeavors which, when undertaken in parallel, will both reinforce the commitment within ourselves and speed up the process of making untainted food as accessible to us in the future as junk food is now.

As we've seen, we have been depleting the soil and it is coming back to haunt us through depleted nutritional levels of our conventional fruits and vegetables. We have been treating our livestock as if they were industrial goods, nothing more than a ball valve or an elbow fitting to be churned out by the millions in the cheapest possible way, and it is coming back to haunt us as mad cow disease, as rampant salmonella, E. Coli outbreaks, Avian flu.

We've been strewing toxins into the air, the soil, the waters and now unprecedented numbers of our children live with asthma, cancers, illnesses of all kinds, illnesses unheard of fifty years ago. Our children, all the world's children, are the only insurance policy humankind has.

Our current status quo is undermining their ability to reproduce, their ability to think clearly, and their ability to protect themselves, not from foreign threats, but from corporate fascism and corporate oligarchy, from greed.

We realize that we must acknowledge our place in the cycle of all things –earth, animals, birds, insects and other human beings– or we cannot expect the very basics of health and safety for ourselves or our offspring. You *get* that the treachery and malaise that has been wreaked on the planet in the last 70 years can only begin to be undone if each of us decides to forgo the convenience and the chemicals that the Big Ag/ Pharmaceutical conglomerates insist we need. And so, you've made a decision: to eat more simply, more conscientiously; to eat food that is as pure as you can find.

You have made a choice that will help humankind turn a corner in history. We can put the brakes on incipient climate changes, slow or reverse the decimation of other species, and most importantly, put an end to the obesity, illness, pharmaceutical dependence and much of the self-induced mental havoc of our own species. We can only do it by learning to worship our food.

Only in recognizing that the integrity of our DNA -our cells, our organ systems, our very being- is dependent upon the food that we eat, can we once again begin to revere the source of all that we are. And all that we are is all that is around us, growing and living. Forget the pipe dream of earlier generations– that when we "used up" the resources of the earth we would simply move on to pod colonies on distant planets. People actually believed this. It is not even close to feasible. The fallacy of "Better Living through Chemicals" has also been revealed as, if not a lie, then a wry reminder of the hubris of yesterday's failed dominance/ conquer mentality.

This is it. Reach down and touch the ground, the earth. This is what we have to work with. When we understand clearly that all life here on our planet, discovered and as yet undiscovered, is part of an awesome, interlaced, interdependent world of bacteria, fungi, algae, and energy pulsing through the soil particles, the water droplets of the atmosphere, the forests, fields and the seas, through us, through every creature— a delicate, fragile balance we call Nature —only then can we appreciate the urgency of the changes we still need to make.

There are those who say that it is impossible to feed the entire population of the planet with organically grown food. Even if that were the case, which I do not believe it to be, are you going to be the one who will voluntarily sacrifice yourself and your descendants to the alter of chemical commerce? In other words, knowing that it is the best possible route for the health of your family and future generations of your family to pursue, will you be the one to nonetheless continue to purchase decoy foods for the sake of somebody else's foundering economy? I think not. It is time for a revolution in the way we think and the way we do business.

Food, friends and family are all that we really have. As an era of greed for material goods comes to an end, we'll find that sustenance and sharing are all that really matters. We must work immediately to overcome the conditions that have brought us to a place of complacency or trepidation regarding our grocery choices. Remember, it wasn't simply that these things were offered and we chose them. Our confidence in our own ability to choose was undermined. So, know now that you have the wherewithal to understand what is healthy.

Go back to basics and trust in yourself. Our dreams and ambitions have been depicted as being under threat by advertisements which keep telling us we haven't got enough *stuff*. They show us people just like us (only happier, wealthier, thinner) and we are asked to believe that we can become that, if only we buy, or keep buying ... "X."

Instead, notice for once, not all those who have more comforts, but the leagues of those who have less. Look around you and realize what you already have. Look around at your actual neighbors and realize that your life is not very different from theirs; the people in the ads do not really exist. There are those who have more things, but happier, safer, without tragedy or pain? No one has it all.

Comfort, safety and security are not bought, they are shared. Inner peace isn't purchased at a spa. Inner peace is achieved through the lifelong accumulation of tiny joys. And those joys are acquired like small sparks of electricity, one at a time, through the act of touching, of reaching out, of giving. Without deliberation or intention, you one day find that are being warmed by the spark you gave, the exchange of energy you offered.

If you really want to feel fulfilled, to distract yourself from the boredom that induces you to eat, if you want to find something else to think about besides the latest diet fad or how you look, there are (in English) three words that will help you get there.

They form a phrase common to some of the longest lived people in all cultures. These three words have been spoken stoically by withered matriarchs with heads held high, and whispered through gritted teeth by mothers wracked by accident or disease. The phrase has been murmured by some of the worlds bravest soldiers, and it has kept them all going. It is among the most powerful in any language.

Despite what the 1980's may have led you to believe, contrary to what the marketing mavens or the entire field of feel-good professionals bent on pampering for profit has told you for the last 30 years, the phrase is not "I deserve it."

The three most important words are, "They need me."

You are needed. You may not even know by whom yet, but you are needed. There are myriad ways we can make a difference in the lives of those around us, all of them important. It is time for us to rebuild a connectedness, not just within families but with all those around us who are a part of what makes up the network of our community.

This isn't a check-writing experience, this is where you give of your time. The benefit that you will reap will far outweigh the expenditure. The changes in your own life will be incalculable.

Your children may already seem like a full-time job, precluding you from reaching out to others, but what better opportunity for them to gain the rewards of giving in their own lives than to accompany you in your selfless acts? Your job may be consuming, but is it fulfilling? It may offer prestige, it may bring you material goods, but unless you are helping others, there is something missing and you feel it.

Give up the golf game and get your buddies together to repair the porch of your elderly neighbors. Pull on your wellies and clean a local stream or river bank. Forgo the weekly manicure and create a visiting reading group in which members read aloud to residents at senior homes, hospices or hospitals. They will ask about your new stainless-steel lunch pail, you will explain about your commitment to healthier eating and a healthier world and another spark will flicker, lighting the way to a larger movement. That's how it happens, it's that simple.

We make these connections because we are grateful. Grateful that we have the opportunity to build a 4' square, raised garden bed in our yard and watch organic vegetables bloom from the earth. Grateful that we have our family (be it a biological bond or a family created through bonds of love.) Grateful for our friends, our youth, our health or even just a roof over our heads. Grateful enough to want to share.

People around the country have begun to reinstitute the concept of tithing into their lives. Most religious groups require this in the form of donation, and that is fine; the tithing I refer to is not in the form of finance, but a gift of yourself. This is you being present. Giving back is coming back into fashion. In a renaissance of the tribal cultures of our ancestors, let the measure of your wealth be the extent of your reach in giving.

Can you volunteer to cook once a month at a local shelter? Can you deliver food to the homebound? Maybe what these associations need is a delivery of healthy organic vegetables from your garden, or a portion of the certified grassfed meat that you sell? How extraordinary to be able to pass on, not just your conviction in the benefits of real, wholesome food, but the food itself.

There are many communities around the country who have begun to establish *Plant a Row for the Hungry* programs to make it easy for farmers and even gardeners to contribute their excess produce to those who really need it. This program was started by the Garden Writers Association and many towns and cities already have in place organizations willing to accept food, and lists of vegetables that are needed to be grown. See about starting your own chapter if there isn't one nearby.

Maybe your local school cafeteria would benefit from a gift of your garden's bounty, contact them at the start of growing season to see what foods might help. Many school districts are beginning to suffer from the financial crisis blighting municipalities across the country. Cutting back on quality food for our children –and all children are our children– is not a direction we can allow them to take.

Maybe you have the time to organize local gardeners who might want to join you in donating to the school district. Perhaps you would even consider organizing a group to create a garden at the local school, which, with the help of teachers and even students themselves, could become a learning tool as well as a source of nutrition. Depending on the size of the school, a student club could be created, lesson plans could use the garden as a jumping off point for math, science, or other fields (What is the Latin name of the plant? What does it mean? How did it get that name? What is its name in Spanish/ French/ Ethiopian/ Hmong? Is the meaning different?)

A garden can be used to learn about cultural diversity—grow foods eaten by as many ethnic backgrounds as are represented in the school. Learn how to cook dishes made with those foods. Can't commit to something that consuming? How about making a meal once a month for the elderly widower at the end of the block?

Our own neighborhoods, our own cities and towns can once again become a source of the many small acts that bring true comfort. We must work hard to overcome the isolation we have been made to feel regarding our community. In rural areas people commonly connect for an hour or so on Sunday mornings, but this time is focused on a minister, not on interactivity. Our workdays are consumed with solitary activities for most adults, whether this means a cash register, a cubicle, a place on the assembly line, a tractor seat or the transporting of young ones from place to place. Rarely will today's work environment require us to work as a team, despite the endless use of cloying corporate inanities like "team player."

Urban lives, while more congested, are typically even more insular- ever changing faces at the shops, (the shops themselves seem to change from day to day,) subways or streets a blur of humanity, our vehicles each a discrete bubble shut off from one another. The simple recognition of a familiar vendor at a newsstand kiosk can feel like a welcome bond. The divide and conquer tactics of modern marketing —of seeing the Joneses as the bar against which to measure ourselves rather than seeing them as extra hands to rely upon during the harvest— have cost us dearly.

We must slow our pace, not just in food but in life. It is time to make time for a deeper connection with those around us; sharing a goal of creating a saner world is a good place to start. What this also means is overcoming the sense of competition so many feel about every aspect of our lives. Auspiciously, by making inroads in either of these directions we benefit ourselves as well.

We need to begin to engage in a fully conscious life, it isn't enough to give lip service to environmental crisis, or to Paypal a donation while sustaining a lifestyle flagrantly at odds with our professed goals. Working to guarantee that all people have access to quality food free from contaminants is the only way to assure that *we* will continue to have it. And it is a hands-on endeavor. The good news is that more and more people are making this commitment. A way to expedite the process of finding access to healthier, toxin-free lives is to connect with groups or organizations already working towards this goal. There is such a groundswell of activity in this country right now that there's virtually no region where some type of gathering isn't already underway.

Look around, often like-minded people come in different shapes, sizes, ages, colors and backgrounds from what we are expecting.

Likewise, our pursuit may not follow the path that we'd envisioned. Follow your gut and see where it takes you. Getting engaged in your community can mean many things. The organizations you join do not always have to involve food directly- maybe you will be the one sharing insights and inciting new enterprises with friends you've made through other activities.

The secret is to find a gathering in which everyone interacts. The options are as varied as the people interested. There are activities which involve food— a weekly or monthly dinner club where participants rotate between houses, sharing not only dishes, but intentionally working together in the creation of those dishes.

Time is spent intertwined in the spirit of the tamaladas mentioned in chapter four, the Cajun shellfish boil, or a Chinese community stir-fry where everybody brings an ingredient, or, along those same lines, the evening could be a "Stone Soup" gathering or a pizza making event. Men alongside women can be encouraged to engage in the cooking or prep; children as well. TVs must remain off, story-telling or singing rules the day. Eating is *not* the main activity— the production, the preparation, the weaving of yarns and building of history together is the focal point of the afternoon or evening. Eating is the winding down. As others have said, it's about the journey.

Creating rituals in which we assist others can become an annual part of a family's traditions. I have another sister who uses the time between Thanksgiving and Christmas to have her children choose toys from their closets and toy boxes to donate to needy children. The custom can be established to include one toy or many dolls, games and gadgets, but must be things of value and not dirty or broken.

For one week, starting the Saturday after Thanksgiving Day, toys are debated and inspected, gathered and maybe even wrapped. (The Sunday comics are a good, non-commercial wrapping paper.) The emphasis is that this is a gift and it would cause disgrace and embarrassment to the gift-giver if the item were shoddy or second-rate. If your child is of an appropriate age, attending the event and giving the gift to someone who is delighted by it can be a heartwarming experience that he or she will want to re-create.

Another idea gaining great popularity is community gardening. A plot of land, a little bit of organizing and suddenly people you would never have gotten to know are sharing their grandmother's tips for ridding the garden of snails (as long as it doesn't involve synthetic pesticides!) and helping you carry that second bushel of cucumbers to your car.

Gardens not only provide a place to engage with other people, they are an excellent way to reignite an awe for the magic of life's cycles. Whether musing over an entire wheelbarrow of pumpkins propagated from a single seed or contemplating a bushel of green beans sprung forth from a tiny bean, gardeners of all ages find wonder in the miracle of life's renewal. Gardening can also mean a modest amount or a great deal of exercise, depending on what you put into it. It can be an endless opportunity for learning for children, an occasion of meditative productivity for elderly folks, and best of all, you can eat the results of all your hard work. Nothing tastes better on a warm sunny day than a sweet juicy strawberry you have grown yourself.

If you can't find communal space for a true community garden, consider a new kind of garden club: by pre-arranged agreement, you grow a few vegetables in your yard and several neighbors, or other-moms-of-third-graders, or little league dads, all chose to grow different vegetables and herbs. During harvest seasons you get together once a week to share and trade. Everybody could grow a component of salsa for instance - tomatoes, cilantro, onions, various chilies. Or you could agree to grow things that are ready to be harvested at different times-someone grows cantaloupes, someone grows corn, someone grows potatoes.

Of course, no one ever wants to grow only one thing, so there will undoubtedly be rosemary and borage and yellow squash and mint with which to surprise your friends. As resources in some communities may become a bit stretched in these difficult economic times, the sharing of food can be a valuable way include fresh local organic variety in the evening meal without the costs associated if those same foods purchased were from a retail outlet. More importantly, it provides an opportunity for good fellowship and the pleasure of not toiling alone.

Even if gardening is not something you choose to participate in as a group or social activity, everyone should find a way to begin to grow at least some of their own foods. The rewards are immeasurable. Food is only one facet of the merits of gardening.

The connection with nature, understanding the soil as a living ecosystem, appreciating the contributions of fungi and earthworms and beneficial insects to our environment, to our lives, these things can once again provide the awareness and respect for seasons, rain, and sunshine, that so many in our culture have lost. A 2008 study done at the University of Michigan showed that even a modest interaction with nature can improve both mood and brain function.[1]

At the very least if you can manage nothing else, a renewed relationship with food and creation can be had in something as simple as a small pot on your windowsill. Grow parsley or lemon thyme. Learn to use them. Grow oregano or mint or tiny peppers.

Whatever you choose, do it without the "miracle" growing powders and liquids, the "wonder" garden chemicals, the "just this once" applications of insect poisons and weed killers. Be sure not to start potted plants with chemically treated potting soil, don't add anything but natural augmentation to your garden.

You can do it. Things will grow just as they did for hundreds of thousands of years before toxic synthetic chemicals seeped into our lives. They say you can't feed the world that way, but remember, you aren't feeding the world, you are just feeding you. And a few friends.

Celebration

Now, as in the past, where there is sharing, there is celebration. Every culture around the world includes food at some point during their celebrations. In contrast, in American culture today the feast is nearly the only aspect of our celebrations that we have retained. Feasting, and a lemming-like drive to purchase whatever kibble the retailers have deemed essential to the season: chocolate for Valentine's Day, more chocolate for Easter, fireworks for the Fourth of July, candy of every stripe for Halloween, more candy for Christmas or Hanukkah.

Worse, in the last several decades it seems we are supposed to purchase endless ornamentation for our homes, our yards, our person, often going so far as to necessitate new table decorations, new place settings, even new window treatments and lawn litter for holidays as minor as Valentine's Day, Halloween or the Fourth of July. In fact, the acquisition of schlock has come to supercede even the food component of most of our holidays in economic terms.

The original Thanksgiving was very much about gratitude and prayer. (And, needless to say, not at all about watching football.) Yule, the precursor to Christmas, involved much singing and dancing along with rituals both solemn and frivolous to assure a safe, fruitful new year. Parades, songs, bodily adornment, time honored rites, conventions and traditions, often with spiritual significance, make up the festivities of many older cultures. One major aspect of the yearly observances in nearly all peoples around the world is fasting.

Most societies observe some kind of fasting, usually related to spiritual practices. Nearly every religion has evolved holidays or celebrations employing hallowed rites enacted around ritualistic fasting. Fasting for an entire day, (I don't recommend fasting from water, but only food) serves the purpose of putting one's life into perspective. In most situations, this is aided by a meditation of some kind, often, when words are used, this is called prayer.

I suggest that we rekindle the practice of fasting, not only individually, but as a national observation. One day a year could be set aside for all Americans to reflect upon our wealth and good fortune. No food is eaten throughout the day (by those adults healthiest enough to participate) though non-alcoholic beverages, including healthy smoothies for those unaccustomed to fasting, are encouraged.

It is a day spent engaged in activities which will impact others outside the home, however projects can take place at home or within the community.

It could be quite rewarding to create elaborate rituals from scratch. The day could begin within the home in a shared song of thankfulness to the farmers who provide our food. Each member of the family or group of friends could gather at the usual meal time and speak one line of indebtedness towards a food that is missing from that day, an aspect of the process of preparing that food, an animal on which we humans are dependent, the wind, the water or any and all of the incalculable facets of our meals.

The lighting of candles, pre-determined periods of silent reflection and gratitude, these are features of fasting in many cultures. Our holiday could choose a time of day, say three o'clock in the afternoon, to be spent in a collective ritual of remembrance of and unity with the rest of the world: one candle lit per group, and a nationwide thirty minutes of sedentary silence observed.

A gentle afternoon hike could be planned, or some other respite into nature, a park, a waterfront; not strenuous or competitive, but reflective, pleasant, playful. There are no cards, no gifts, no gear needed on this holiday, its sentiment comes from the profound recognition of our place in the tapestry of nature, and our ties to each other. At sunset a modest meal is shared: a light soup, some homemade bread and tea.

In the evening, members of the family or gathering could share readings of current or historical events about others who do not have access to the bounty that we have, to reinforce our comprehension of the plenitude that most of us in the Western world have. Stories could be created imagining one's self in the circumstances of someone in a refugee camp or a city under trade sanctions. Plans could be devised about ways to help, or shared about the ways in which each member is already engaged in helping alleviate the hunger of others.

During the rest of the year, personal fasting is something individuals could consider as a way of examining their relationship with abundance. We are unaccustomed to depriving ourselves, yet many cultures with far less in the way of material comforts regularly practice physical deprivation as a way of learning self-discipline and understanding sacrifice.

A fast can take many forms. It can be the removal of one food for a period of time as in Lenten practices. It can be the intentional missing of a particular meal. It can mean eating nothing from sunrise until sunset or depriving oneself of all food for a 24 hour period or longer. Fasting, in addition to the spiritual benefit it provides, can be another way of understanding and reinforcing the value of the food that we regularly do eat.

If you do decide you want to try fasting, there are some things to consider. Plan your fast. Have a list of activities to engage in, step outside your usual routine. Give yourself choices. Direct your activity outward. Make this a time you consider the less fortunate in the world, people who are often hungry. Make this a time you collect cans or clothes for the local women's shelter. Make this a time you work on that part of your garden that you've dedicated to the local senior center, and whose bounty you will deliver to them all summer.

Perhaps this could be a time that you could volunteer at a local soup kitchen, growing in yourself not only by serving but in being around food that you choose not to eat, knowing that if you did it would take that meal from someone more needy.

When you fast, notice the feeling of hunger. Examine it the way a blind child might investigate an unfamiliar object. Explore its edges; learn not to be afraid of it. In the past you may have interpreted this feeling as anxiety, restlessness, irritability. It may have stressed you to find yourself physically craving something and you'd have quickly muted the feeling with food.

In the past, if you'd tried to skip a meal as some form of diet you might have focused inward, engulfed in self pity. You may have felt that you were missing out on something that everyone else was getting, and gone into a self-negating session whose outcome only spiraled you to more indulgence in things that were "bad" for you as self-punishment and further self-victimization. This is different.

Now you know that you are the agent of this feeling. This hunger is intentional. You are in control of it. Grow in your understanding of yourself by learning to understand the sensation of hunger. Feel the strength it builds within you. It makes you want to be active. It is natural that the feeling of hunger would make us want to be active, our early ancestors would have needed that motivation to hunt their next meal. So, you feel restless. This is as it should be.

Use the feeling. Move around. Maybe this is a good time to go for a long walk. Find a way to do it. When I worked in an office complex within a wasteland of office complexes, I often walked during my lunch break in lieu of eating. There were no sidewalks, there was no place to *go*. There were several major six-lane highways lined with countless beige and brick warehouse/office buildings, intersected by side roads containing more warehouses.

Trucks roared down these roads helter-skelter, never expecting to encounter someone on foot. It was actually dangerous. I walked anyway. I concentrated on the sunshine, or the brisk air, or the gentle drizzle. (And of course, on not getting run over.) Wear an orange vest if you need to, the important goal is your clear and self-assured focus. Feel yourself tighten your stomach muscles. Feel yourself grow in a potentiality that is outside of food. (And feel relief from the mid-day coma that lunch often brings.)

This is not a power walk. It is not a competition with yourself or others; there is no timer, no stopwatch. It does not require membership, special paraphernalia, or a change of clothes, though a comfortable pair of flat shoes would seem to make sense. Don't be lured into buying anything for this adventure. This walk is a simple, purposeful, unfaltering stride, each step a step into the future, an exploration of the present, a contemplation.

Spend the time considering ways in which you will be an instrument of change in the world. Dream. Visualize. Give yourself at least as much time as it would have taken to amass and consume a meal.

If you are unable to walk for any reason, consider meditation. It isn't necessary to know a chant or even to chant at all, but many people find that it helps with concentration and the ability to tune out external sounds. If you need to, try simply repeating "I am." Breathe. Don't be afraid to move, to rock slowly or sway in a gentle repetitive way; it helps to involve the body as much as possible. In this meditation, as with the walk, allow yourself to think. See in your mind's eye the ways in which you can make a difference.

Children, too, can be encouraged to involve themselves in fasts of various kinds. A child in a strictly observant Catholic household often must chose one favorite item to refrain from eating during the period of Lent. It isn't necessary that this practice be related to the period of Lent or of Catholicism.

A pre-Thanksgiving fast might be developed along these lines wherein one gives up bread or French fries. The choice should be difficult, something regularly encountered and should matter to the child. It is important that the effort and practice be sincere. Naturally, children should not be expected to do this alone, but be invited to join their parent or parents in these exercises.

A family or an individual may choose to eliminate meat from their meals for one day a week (or more) as a form of fasting. With children, this needs to happen in the context of conversation about why this change is taking place and about the importance of our food choices. Feeling a financial pinch? Use this opportunity to examine with the family what other families around the world are experiencing. Your family may choose to refrain from eating one evening meal each month in fellowship with an "adopted" community or a family to whom you donate.

Another type of fast might be to eat only brown rice or a single grain or staple like yucca for a day, in the manner of many poor people around the world. Again, this should invite discussion about those who eat like this most days of the week. It is time to re-instill in our children the concepts of restraint and self-discipline as well as learning about the value of food.

In addition to fasting from food, one evening a month might include "fasting" from all forms of electronic entertainment as well. Quietly reading or better yet, reading out loud to one another could be the evening's entertainment. Singing together is another possibility. Think you can't sing?

Music

Singing and dancing have been integral to every civilization on the planet. Human beings sing as readily and as easily as breathing. In fact, in the Inupiaq language the word breathe is the same as the word for song. And yet most Americans will tell you that they "can't sing." Nearly as many feel uncomfortable dancing, though even tiny infants respond to rhythm with movement— they can't help themselves.

Dancing was once a natural response to happy events, an unbridled expression of joy, exuberance. Now, with the exception of the occasional wedding, or unless you meet up with Ellen DeGeneres, dance has been relegated to the young. Even then, often only to those who are perceived of as bold enough or inebriated enough.

Singing is something many of us feel timid about even as children. This is a staggering tragedy, though one that is not taken seriously. It is a sad truth that, as with so many other capabilities, we have turned over the making of music to "the specialists."

Susan Brink, staff writer for the L.A. Times, describes perfectly the moment for many of us when singing ended:

> IT'S George's fault that I never sang. Freckle-faced, hair-licked, musical-fingered George. Starting in first grade, I sat behind him in the alto row in music class, and that remained my place for eight years of grammar school.
>
> He was Mr. Perfect Pitch, the kid who could play "Flight of the Bumblebee" on the piano. I'd open my mouth to sing, and he'd turn around and snap, "You're flat. You're flat." "I've been workin' on

the railroad...." I'd begin. "You're flat," I'd hear from the seat in front of me. Pretty early on, I learned to lip-sync."[2]

(it's a wonderful article, see chapter 7 citations for link)

Unless you were wise enough, as George obviously was, to have been born into a family of musicians, your early years are often bereft of music, especially the making of music. By the time you enter kindergarten it can become nearly impossible to catch up. Although there are similarities with a child entering a school in which her native language is not spoken, it would be as if no one in the school spoke at all except for one hour a week—and *then* spoke another language. (Many schools no longer even have one hour a week for music class.)

Children who speak the language of music do not realize why someone else stumbles, and like children often do, taunt and tease, or like little George, react with frustrated intolerance. The musical children are seen as having a "natural" talent; everyone else is lumped into the have-nots, and many times these people never open their mouths in song again. It is the equivalent of losing a limb. We learn to compensate, but our lives are always out of balance.

At one time people sang songs daily. Songs and sing-song rhymes were made up for any reason or no reason at all— to pass the time while walking to the fields, while working with one's hands in countless capacities, as a way of retaining one's oral history, for flirting, for worship, for fun.

The previous centuries had professional musicians, of course. Still, before the era of recorded music the average person in this country, as elsewhere, made music. Most people had at least rudimentary skills with some instrument, it was what people did together. Everybody sang.

In many cultures this is still the case. In the summer of 2000, I had the inestimable pleasure of visiting family in Mitchelstown, Ireland. A huge gathering of "found" American relatives were hosted by the descendents of two brothers. We toured the landmarks associated with the Roche family name and were treated to historic sites, castle banquets, brilliant performances of step-dancing, incredible Irish food and drink and regaled with stories from sun up til sundown. But the best part of the whole affair was that all the Irish kinfolk sang.

Whether to pass the time in the hired tour bus as we traveled from site to site, at the pubs of an evening or taking turns throughout the night on the small stage built for the occasion at the farm of Assumpta and Jim, songs were shared by young and old without competition or self-consciousness. Some songs were stories told by an individual, others were grand events where all were encouraged to join in. It was simply a way of having fun. I have seen this same assembled *joie de vive* in movies and documentaries from Romania, France, South Africa and elsewhere; the film *Since Otar Left*, out of Tbilisi, Georgia, has a wonderful scene of a party with all generations singing familiar songs together. This is not the experience of most Americans.

Singing has been proven to lower blood pressure, to boost the immune system, to calm, soothe, and restore the spirits of nearly everyone who's been studied.[3] It has been suggested that singing regularly in a social gathering, whether it be an casual jam of amateurs or a formal choral group, can even prolong your life. It is an intuitive, primal remedy for healing.

When we sing we are not just creating an auditory experience, our bodies are actually resonating the sounds. In a recent European study, elderly members of a chorus reported "improved lung capacity, high energy, relieved asthma, better posture, and enhanced feelings of relaxation, mood, and confidence after joining the group. Seventy-nine percent felt less stressed, and 75 percent experienced heightened adrenaline and wakefulness after singing."[4]

Singing has been shown to help school age children do better academically, gain focus and direction, and even to help overcome shyness and stuttering. It provides seniors with improved stamina, memory and mental acuity.

Among Alzheimer's patients able to participate in singing groups as a form of treatment, researchers found a renewed ability to engage with others. Patients particularly enjoyed singing, and remembering, songs from their youths. The satisfaction of being able to join the crowd reawakened confidence and played a huge role in elevating mood. Singing ties us to our past, to happier times (not the least because singing itself makes us happier) and to other people, cutting through the barriers of language or politics. Speaking is a prosaic act of communication, singing is the exultation of our humanity to the universe.

Dance is also something that is used therapeutically to comfort and revitalize the elderly, or to bring purpose and possibility to the young. Yet rarely do adults dance once we leave our teens and early twenties. In our increasingly mechanized society it is one of the childish things we put away as we become adults. It seems there isn't time.

Needless to say, there is no common forum for "clap and stomp" in our culture. It is amusing to think of dance being a pre-requisite to a city council meeting or a conference or convention: a rousing Patsch Tants or Moribayassa would not only get our hearts pumping, there would undoubtedly be more accord and less adversity in our workaday dealings.

We need to dance as much as we need to sing. Dance is to our body as dreaming is to our minds. The motion of our bodies flowing in a rhythmic pattern is both soothing and invigorating. It assuages an innate yearning for rhythm within us. This is why hand drumming, particularly with a crowd of drummers or several large drums played with sticks or mallets is such an unforgettable experience. The vibrations reverberate through us, we reverberate with the sound. It is not about just listening to music, as when we sit under headphones lost in sound and segregated from the world (though this can have its place.) It is the participation in music which is vital.

Dancing, not only the movement of our own bodies but the synchronization of ourselves with many people together, is a reinforcement of the primal solace of being part of something larger. For while singing and dancing can each be done alone, the most salubrious, rewarding, enjoyable aspects of these activities occurs when they are done in fellowship with others.

The idea, first proposed several hundred years ago, that man is nothing more than a machine has been one of the most detrimental concepts ever foisted upon the human race. The embodiment of that philosophy has been the industrialization our societies. First the mechanization of people in the industry of manufacturing, and then in the military, the service industry and finally the corporate worlds has left us with the sense that we are interchangeable cogs whether it be the firing line, the assembly line or the office hierarchy. Reducing an individual to an indistinguishable unit of commerce is a deleterious mindset whether it involves cattle or communities.

We seek medication for our antsy-ness, our anxiety, our ADHD. There are dozens of drugs for depression. Looking at the numbers of drugs ingested, both recreationally and as prescribed medications, it could be argued that our society is one of the most mentally disconsolate in all of history. Unlike past cultures, we rarely walk hand-in-hand or arm-in-arm with friends; we avoid touching. We have lost the song and dance "limbs" of our expressive capacity.

By any analysis, the vast apparatus of industry would certainly benefit by eliminating variables like emotion from hirelings in the workplace. It's why the idea of robots is ever so appealing to employers. Barring robots, if the populace could only be kept just a little sick, slightly exhausted, but well enough to continue "going through the motions" of our jobs without complaint or question, the grand commercial industrial pharmaceutical complex would churn on to benefit the vested interest of the few.

So we are encouraged to cling to the belief that we can simply tweak a chemical formula here or there and pop it in our mouths whether we call it food or medicine, and keep the ol' machine (our bodies) running. We likewise holdfast in our minds to the oft-reiterated myth of the individualist, the every-man-for-himself lone pioneer. (Yet who but industry benefits from the kind of opaqueness that prevents us from knowing, for instance, another's salary?) Obedient to the ethos of our era, we try to shoulder-down and push through it all alone, without community.

It is time to realize that we are not machines. There exists an unnamed and unacknowledged grace when people share time and work together on goals outside of that for which they are paid. There is alchemy in altruism. We need each other. We need to help one another. We need, not just a partner, we need to be a part of extended family, however conceived — of humanity, of the environment, of the larger fabric of life.

We need the effusion of magic that happens when we intertwine our voices in harmony. We need the jubilant synchronicity of hand-clapping and foot-tapping with our fellow travelers through this life. The inestimable value of these exploits dictates that they should be seen not simply as frivolous pastimes to be pursued when time allows, but as very real ingredients in the maintenance of our health and well-being.

Find your voice. Into the freylakh (the title of this chapter) means "into the joy" in Yiddish. Move yourself into the joy. And then keep moving. Bring others into the joy to move with you.

I was fortunate some years ago to have lived in an area where there was a local musician who gave group classes for adults who had never sung. Like the LA Times writer mentioned earlier, we always suspected that perhaps we really could sing, had always wanted to try, but had been intimidated by being surrounded by those who might be unwilling to tolerate our learning process.

In a fortuitous experience I found a place where, for a nominal fee, we fledgling singers with no expectation or desire to "go pro," gathered weekly and learned to unkink our rusty vocal chords. In an uncritical setting with much laughter and camaraderie, we learned to sing first through breathing exercises and holding notes, then simple rounds and eventually harmonies. Real harmonies! For our final class, just before a wonderful potluck dinner, we performed for ourselves and those friends and family members who wanted to attend. We sounded great.

The teacher who held these classes gave them several times a year, for years, with groups of 10-15. Though some were more experienced, most who took the workshop had never sung outside of the shower. The class was not one of actual vocal training, and didn't dwell on the nuances of music theory or operatic pronunciations. It was just a place for all ages to free our stifled voices. There were always students.

I would like to see this kind of gathering blossom. This is a call out to musicians all over the country, don't just perform for us, lead us in song. Perhaps all the "little Georges" could begin to make amends. Create an opportunity for bonding, for getting to know local people in an invariably enjoyable environment. These are the settings where like-minded passions are fostered. Here is where you'll find cohorts for your community garden or learn of a source for raw milk.

Before we leave the topic of song, I want to make another suggestion. We need songs for the organic, sustainable food movement. There has never been a movement without song, whether we talk about the anti-Vietnam war movement or the French Revolution, the American revolution, the Civil Rights movement or the various worker's movements throughout history. It is a vital part of our cohesion that we share simple, easily memorized, sing-able songs. So I hereby put out a call to all musicians, writers and song crafters: Please contribute to getting the word out! Help us to support organic, healthy foods in a sustainable, environmentally and community friendly fashion. Write songs! And most importantly, write songs that everybody can sing.

Now, I am a firm believer in the grassroots credo which states that one should not make a suggestion without being willing to act on it themselves. Know that I am not a songwriter, nor do I have any musical training whatsoever. But in the spirit of fun, and in furthering the gaiety to be had pursuing healthy eating, singing and community, I have written three songs which I have contributed to the appendix of this book. Try 'em out. And if I can do it, you can too. So even if you're not a songwriter either, give it a whirl, see what you come up with and share your song with family and friends. It could catch on.

In this same jocular atmosphere, let us remember that old dictum "Laughter is the best medicine." A study conducted by the University of Frankfurt found that belly laughter, the kind that uses your whole diaphragm (like when you're laughing so hard you're gasping for air) is a wonderful tonic for the lymphatic system.[5] Laugh at yourself. Find time to let go of the seriousness of life, no matter how oppressive it seems. Being an adult doesn't mean being dour, rigid, self-flagellating. It means feeling the strength and freedom of one's own convictions, nothing more, nothing less. Leave plenty of room for festivity and playfulness.

There is a need for more holidays, more festivals; real ones. Festivals that mean something, even something simple. Reverence and gratitude around our meals should become a given. Rituals can be fashioned to celebrate the earth, the harvest, the coming planting time.

For example, I like to burn the remnants of my plants with a weed burner after the vegetables have been harvested. It kills some of the dormant insects, fights back the ever-present new weed growth, and provides endless hours of entertainment though some might call it work, depending on how you look at it. (Of course, I'm talking about something in the realm of a 1/4 acre garden, not hundreds of acres of land.)

I can easily see this activity involving several friends or families getting together on a damp, non-windy day or succession of days, torching the garden together from one yard to the next at season's end, and following up with a festival feast of the harvest bounty. Let's raise a glass and sing a song to the Weed Dragon.* It's silly, of course. But, I wouldn't let that stop me. Create your own festivities.

[*Naturally, you wouldn't do this in a drought area. Also, before you torch your weeds, be sure to check out what you have growing and whether or not they are edible or worthwhile for tea or tinctures. Lambsquarters is a wonderful "weed" I found in the garden, it tastes better than cooked spinach and contains more vitamins and minerals.

I also found sorrel, a delightful addition to soups and salads all summer long. Dandelion, nettles, all kinds of "weeds" are known to provide more nutrients than many of the vegetables we grow intentionally, without all the labor. Don't let them go to waste.]

One can create personal rituals or holidays within a family or small group which then get passed on and over time become an established part of your community. This is exactly the process that began any of our current holidays. Already many towns and villages set aside a day to celebrate some locally grown product—there are garlic festivals, corn festivals, pumpkin festivals, yam and mushroom festivals. These and others like them are a wonderful touchstone to our agricultural past and we should work to keep them alive, but with a new twist—let's do it without chemicals.

Let's see who can grow the biggest pumpkin without those "plant steroids." After all, how are plant-enhancing drugs given to plants any different from performance-enhancing drugs given to athletes? Let's give awards to those who can get results without cheating. Let's reward those who instead contribute time and devotion, nurture, knowledge and the skin off their knuckles to the quest for quality.

We have the ability to grow enough food to feed the world if we go about it the right way, with a willingness to work at it. Make the choice to let go of the things that don't matter. Live lightly. Laugh. Learn once again to recognize the power-packed nutrient levels of a smaller, but more flavorful fruit or vegetable. The world can no longer afford to be impetuous or purposeless. We have the answer within ourselves, accepting that feels like a sigh of relief.

Reach out to the many others around you who are discovering the same motivation. No more worry and confusion about which of the many voices trying to guide us is the right one. There is only one answer. We are each the incarnation of our future. We are all shepherds.

We must recognize that our food is all we have, and all we are. In every step along the way, from the soil in which it arises it to the soil it becomes, we must be reverent of the miracles of plant and animal life that surround us. The era of greed and decadence is past.

When the time comes that we, as a nation, are known for our humble gratitude for our next meal, our genuine appreciation of the act of meal preparation, our devotion to maintaining the purity of the soil and water of our homeland, and a reverence for the fruits of that land, only then will we have the self-respect and self-discipline to politically address our national epidemic of obesity. But we won't have to.

The first step is realization. The second step is action. And thus, a true grassroots movement has begun to share knowledge, to spread encouragement and to make this dream a reality.

We are on our way. Join us.

We Need Organic Gardens

(To the tune of:
WE NEED A LITTLE CHRISTMAS
From the show "Mame" (1966) (Jerry Herman)

Pull out your wheelbarrow
Put on your gloves, it's time to grab that hoe again
Get out your seed packs
It may be barely Spring, but—let's plant a row again now!...

Because we need organic gardens
Right this very minute
Look at this McNugget
Who could say what's in it?

Yes, we need organic gardens
Right this very minute
Food standards have been getting blurry
Monsanto reigns, we'd better worry

So broadcast the seaweed
Let's feed the soil with all that—good manure again
Give up the fast food
It's time we finally all became mature again now!

For we've grown a little fatter
Grown a little lazy
Grown a little rusty
Got cabin fever crazy
And we need to see tomatoes
Growing in the daisies
Need organic gardens now

Yes, we have to save the soil
Have to save the rivers
Have to build a stronger
Community of givers
And, we need to see the 'happy'
That only health delivers
We need organic gardens now!

The Vendor's Song

Oh, Louise aims to please with her beans and her flowers
Her smile undaunted in sunshine or showers
Every week morning her baskets she'll fill
To share her good luck and goodwill

(she sings) Green beans, fresh from the garden
Green beans, the best in the land
Green beans, fresh from the garden
Picked by my very own hand

Now Billie and Berta both bring bags of butterbeans
Susy has tote bags and hats like you've never seen
And Judy and Beau with Austin in tow, bring bushels
Of everything green

(they sing) Green beans, fresh from the garden
Green beans, the best in the land
Green beans, fresh from the garden
Picked by my very own hand

And Janna brings eggplant and squash and potatoes
And cukes and zucchinis, four kinds of tomatoes
And conserves and jellies and pickles and peas
[inhale, pause for effect]
And everyone sings with Louise

(they sing) Green beans, fresh from the garden
Green beans, the best in the land
Green beans, fresh from the garden
Picked by my very own hand

[again!...]
Green beans, fresh from the garden
Green beans, the best in the land
Green beans, fresh from the garden
Picked by my very own hand

A waltz.   The Vendor's Song © Quinn Montana 2008

Down to the Market

(to the tune of: "As I Went Down to the River," traditional song)

As I went down to the Market for peas
Studyin' about health and disease
And who provides my groceries
Good lord show me the way!

(chorus:)
Oh sisters let's go down,
let's go down, c'mon down
C'mon sisters, let's go down
To the Farmer's Market for peas

As I went down to the market for greens
Studyin' about economies
And who shall own the soil and seeds
Good lord!   Show me the way

Oh, brothers let's go down...
Etc... (rest of chorus... /brothers...)
To the Farmer's Market for greens

As I went down to the market for beets
Studyin' about technologies
Of herbicides and new "GE"s
Good lord ...show me the way

Oh, mothers let's go down...
Etc... (rest of chorus... /mothers...)
To the Farmer's Market for beets

As I went down to the market for meat
Studyin' about the ways and means
Of industry monopolies...
Good lord show me the way

Oh, fathers let's go down...
Etc... (rest of chorus... /fathers...)
To the Farmer's Market for meat

As I went down to the market for treats
Studyin' about the honey bees
and pesticide catastrophes
Good lord show me the way

Oh, neighbors let's go down...
Etc... (rest of chorus... /neighbors...)
To the Farmer's Market for treats

(Final repeat without verse) —
Oh, neighbors let's go down...
Etc...
To our Farmer's Market to eat!

Lyrics © Quinn Montana 2008

Here's to Your Health!

Appendix II

Citations, Chapter 1—

1. Linda S. Kantor, Kathryn Lipton, Alden Manchester, and Victor Oliveira. "Estimating and Addressing America's Food Losses." Food Review, Jan-Apr 1997, p. 3, http://www.ers. usda.gov/Publications/FoodReview/Jan1997/Jan97a.pdf

    "USDA's Economic Research Service (ERS) recently undertook a review of the current data on food waste and built on this knowledge to generate new estimates of food loss by food retailers (supermarkets, convenience stores, and other retail outlets), and consumers and foodservice establishments (storage, preparation, and plate waste in households and foodservice establishments).

    These losses were estimated by applying known waste factors, gathered from published studies and discussions with commodity experts, to the amount of edible food available for human consumption in the United States. However, losses of nonedible food parts such as bones, pits, seeds, and peels, were excluded.

    According to the new (1997)** ERS estimates, about 96 billion pounds of food, or 27 percent of the 356 billion pounds of the edible food available for human consumption in the United States, were lost to human use at these three marketing stages in 1995. ERS does not know the share of these losses that are recoverable.

    However, we can get an idea of the significance of loss by calculating the potential benefit of recovery. On average, each American consumes about 3 pounds of food each day. If even 5 percent of the 96 billion pounds were recovered, that quantity would **represent the equivalent of a day's food for each of 4 million people.** Recovery rates of 10 percent and 25 percent would provide enough food for the equivalent of 8 million and 20 million people, respectively.

    The loss estimates presented here are tentative and are intended to serve as a starting point for additional research. Many of the studies on which these estimates are based date from the mid-1970's or before."

    *Note: There are 70 countries out of 192, with pop. less than 4 mil. [http://worldatlas.com/aatlas/populations/ctypopls.htm]

    **This figure most likely saw a vast increase in the ensuing decade.

2. Ibid., 2.

3. Tom Philpott. "How the feds make bad-for-you food cheaper than healthful fare." Grist, posted 10:46 pm on 22 Feb 2006, retrieved November 2007 http://www.grist.org/news/maindish/2006/02/22/philpott/

4. Howard Lyman. McLibel 2, Produced and directed by Franny Armstrong, 1994. Mr. Lyman was interviewed by One-Off Productions, 1 April 1996; McSpotlight: original transcripts, http://www.mcspotlight.org/

5. S&S Labs. Strasburger and Seigel, Inc., Food testing laboratories, 2003-2006, http://www.sas-labs.com/general/glossary.asp

6. Union of Concerned Scientists. "They Eat What? The Reality of Feed at Animal Factories." Food & Agriculture, Last Revised: 08/08/06, retrieved January 2008 http://www.ucsusa.org/food_and_agriculture/science_and_impacts/impacts_industrial_agriculture/they-eat-what-the-reality-of.html

7. Michael Pollen. "Industrial Corn." Omnivore's Dilemma, (New York; Penguin Press, 2006), p. 15-119

8. Shereen Mahnami, Kathleen Bertolani. KETCHUM Public Relations, for California Dried Plum Board, February 27, 2006, retrieved November 2007 http://www.tummywise. com/release_survey.php

9. Bryan Vartabedian. "Gastroesophageal Reflux Disease Escalating in Children." Nov 1, 2007, http://parentingsolved.typepad.com/parenting_solved/reflux_colic/page/2/. He is quoting reflux epidemiologist Dr. Susan Nelson of Northwestern University who spoke at the North American Society of Pediatric Gastroenterology, Hepatology and Nutrition in Salt Lake City in 2007, retrieved December 2007

10. Organic Consumers Association. "Background Information on Ingredients in So-Called "Natural" BodyCare Products." Retrieved April 2008 http://www.organicconsumers.org/ bodycare/natural_bodycare_ingredients.cfm

11. Cornell Cooperative Extension. "Genetically Engineered Foods in the Marketplace." Genetically Engineered Organisms Public Issues Education (GEO-PIE) Project, July 5, 2001, v1.0, retrieved January 2007 http://www.geo-pie.cornell.edu/educators/downloads/ flier1.pdf

12. Mary Vance Terrain. "The Dark Side of Soy." Utne Reader, July / August 2007, p.2, retrieved August 2007 http://www.utne.com/2007-07-01/TheDarkSideofSoy.aspx?page=2

13. Reference for Business, Encyclopedia of American Industries. "Pesticides And Agricultural Chemicals, Not Elsewhere Classified." Heading: Industry leaders, 2007, retrieved August 2007 http://www.referenceforbusiness.com/industries/Chemicals-Allied/ index.html

14. Alan Greene, MD. "Dr. Greene Content, Dr. Greene's Organic Rx -- Item #9." March 8, 2007, retrieved August 2007 http://www.drgreene.com/21_2163.html

15. John Henkel. "Soy: Health Claims for Soy Protein, Questions About Other Components." FDA Consumer magazine, May-June 2000, retrieved February 2008 http://www.fda.gov/ Fdac/features/2000/300_soy.html

16. Robert Herron, PhD. "Banned PCBs and agrochemicals in blood reduced 50% by centuries-old detoxification procedure." Townsend Letter for Doctors and Patients, Health Industry, bnet, 2002; retrieved May 2008 http://findarticles.com/p/articles/mi_m0ISW/ is_2002_Nov/ai_93736383/

17. Wikipedia: Archer Daniels Midland. Retrieved January 2008 http://en.wikipedia.org/ wiki/Archer_Daniels_Midland

18. Donald L. Barlett And James B. Steele, "Monsanto's Harvest of Fear." Vanity Fair, May 2008, p. 2, retrieved June 2008 http://www.vanityfair.com/politics/features/2008/05/ monsanto200805?currentPage=2

19. Pesticide Action Network North America (PANNA), "World-wide regulatory status of endosulfan." 2008, retrieved June 2008 http://www.panna.org/node/1686

20. Alexis Madrigal. "Give Thanks? Science Supersized Your Turkey Dinner." Wired, November 25, 2008; retrieved November 2008 http://blog.wired.com/ wiredscience/2008/11/turkeytech.html

21. National Men's Resource Center, "High Fructose Corn Syrup." Menstuff, 1996-2004, http://www.menstuff.org/issues/byissue/highfructose.html , sourced from: Wise Traditions in Food, Farming and the Healing Arts, the quarterly magazine of the Weston A. Price Foundation, Fall 2001; retrieved February 2008 www.westonaprice.org/motherlinda/ cornsyrup.html

22. Rich Murray. "How Aspartame Became Legal - The Timeline." From Norfolk Genetic

Appendix II

Information Network (Taken from Welcome to the Spin Machine by Michael Manville http://www.freezerbox.com/archive/2001/04/biotech/ http://www.freezerbox.com/) The Aspartame/NutraSweet Timeline, http://www.swankin-turner.com/aspartame.html by James Turner, ESQ. Director of the National Institute of Science, Law, and Public Policy (NISLAPP) National Institute of Science, Law, and Public Policy 1400 16th Street, NW, Suite 330, Washington, DC 20036 nislapp@swankin-turner.com, December 2002, retrieved November 2006 http://www.rense.com/general33/legal.htm

23. Susan Enfield Esrey. "Organic matters." Delicious Living, Sep 1, 2007, retrieved September 2007. http://deliciouslivingmag.com/greenliving/dl_article_2379/

24. Healthy Child Healthy World. "Quick Tips: 10 Fruits and Vegetables to Buy Organic." HCHW, Live Healthy, retrieved October 2007, http://healthychild.org/live-healthy/ checklist/10_fruits_and_vegetables_to_buy_organic/

25. Charlotte Hartman. Press Release, The National Sludge Alliance, October 15, 2001, http:// www.riles.org/NSA.htm; also see: Duff Wilson, "Fear In The Fields -- How Hazardous Wastes Become Fertilizer." Seattle Times, Business: Thursday, July 03, 1997, retrieved August 2007 http://seattletimes.nwsource.com/news/special/fear_fields.html

26. Siri Nilsson. "Viral Meat Spray: Advancing Food Safety?" ABC News Medical Unit, Sept. 19, 2006, retrieved October 2006 http://abcnews.go.com/Health/ Story?id=2464943&page=1

27. Delthia Ricks. "Spray to quell E. coli: Baltimore company seeking FDA approval for viral substance to kill the bacteria on produce, raw meat." Newsday, April 23, 2007, retrieved August 2007 http://www.intralytix.com/Intral_News_amNewYork.htm

28. Wikipedia: Cell Nucleus. Retrieved October 2006. http://en.wikipedia.org/wiki/Cell_nucleus

29. Robert F. Service. SCIENCE POLICY: Priorities Needed for Nano-Risk Research and Development, News Focus, Science 6 October 2006: Vol. 314. p. 45

30. Etc Group, "Nano's Troubled Waters: Latest toxic warning shows nanoparticles cause brain damage in aquatic species and highlights need for a moratorium on the release of new nanomaterials." Genotype, Thursday, 1 April 2004, retrieved October 2006. http:// www.etcgroup.org/upload/publication/116/01/gt_troubledwater_april1.pdf

31. Barnaby J. Feder. "Engineering Food at Level of Molecules." New York Times, Technology, October 10, 2006, retrieved October 17, 2006. http://www.nytimes. com/2006/10/10/technology/10nano.html?pagewanted=2&_r=2&ref=technology

32. Nanotechnology White Paper, The Nanotechnology Workgroup, Environmental Protection Agency, Science Policy Council, February 2007, sec. 1.5, p. 18, EPA 100/B-07/001

33. Kevin Maney. "Nanotechnology's everywhere." USA Today, Money, Industries, Technology, 5/31/2005, retrieved October 2007 http://www.usatoday.com/money/ industries/technology/maney/2005-05-31-nanotech_x.htm

34. Environmental Working Group. "Bisphenol A: Toxic Plastics Chemical in Canned Food." A Survey of Bisphenol A in U.S. Canned Foods, March 5, 2007, retrieved October 2007 http://www.ewg.org/reports/bisphenola

35. Dani Veracity. "White Flour Contains Diabetes-Causing Contaminant Alloxan." Natural News.com, June 02, 2005, retrieved September 2006 http://www.naturalnews. com/008191.html

36. Joanna Blythman. "Give us our daily chemicals ..." The Guardian, 18 May 2007, retrieved 9/22/07 http://www.guardian.co.uk/profile/joannablythman

37. Katie Hafner. "Ida R. Hoos Is Dead at 94; a Critic of Systems Analysis." The New York Times, May 5, 2007, http://www.nytimes.com/2007/05/05/us/05hoos.html

38. Organic Consumers Association, "What's Wrong With Food Irradiation." February 2001, retrieved February 2008 http://www.organicconsumers.org/Irrad/irradfact.cfm

39. James Gormley. "Food Irradiation - "Protecting" Us?" Citizens for Health, retrieved 02/24/08, http://www.citizens.org/consumer-corner/food-irradiation-protecting-us

40. Ibid.

41. Mark Radinzel. "Doublespeak and You." Capstone Project: http://marcradinzel.efoliomn. com/index, retrieved February 2008. His information was taken from *Double Speak: How Government, Business Advertisers, and Others use Language to Deceive you* written by William Lutz, Harpercollins (September 1990).

42. Ashley Simmons Hotz. "Poison For Profit", redflagsweekly.com, 15may02, retrieved August 2008 http://www.mindfully.org/Pesticide/2002/Poison-For-Profit15ma02.htm

43. Coming Clean. "What is Body Burden?" Body Burden Home Page. Retrieved 08/04/08, http://www.chemicalbodyburden.org/whatisbb.htm

44. Rod Dreher. "USDA-Disapproved: Small farmers and big government." National Review, Jan 27, 2003, BNET News Publications. Retrieved January 2008 http://findarticles. com/p/articles/mi_m1282/is_1_55/ai_96403711/

45. Philip Brasher. "Scientists Study Possible Link Between Ethanol Byproduct and E. coli." The Des Moines Register, January 28, 2008, retrieved January 2008 http://www. cornucopia.org/2008/01/scientists-study-possible-link-between-ethanol-byproduct-and-e-coli/

46. Stephen J Hedges. "E. coli loophole cited in recalls: Tainted meat can be sold if cooked." The Chicago Tribune, Washington Bureau, November 11, 2007, retrieved January 2008 http://archives.chicagotribune.com/2007/nov/11/food/chi-meat_bdnov11 The agency allows companies to put this E. coli-positive meat in a special category -- "cook only." Cooking the meat, the USDA and producers say, destroys the bacteria and makes it safe to eat as precooked hamburgers, meat loaf, crumbled taco meat and other products.

47. David Suzuki Foundation. "Thinking critically about information sources." September 6, 2000; retrieved February 2008 http://www.davidsuzuki.org/About_us/Dr_David_Suzuki/ Article_Archives/weekly09060001.asp

  "A 247 page report recently released by the World Health Organization (WHO), details how tobacco companies have systematically sought to undermine WHO's research and efforts to curb tobacco use for more than a decade.

  Tactics used by the tobacco companies included paying WHO employees to spread misinformation, hiring institutions and individuals to discredit the WHO, secretly funding reports designed to distort scientific studies and even covertly monitoring WHO meetings and conferences.

  Confidential tobacco company documents do not mince words as to the industry's goals, using phrases like: "Discredit key individuals," "Attack WHO," and "Work with journalists to question WHO priorities, budget, role in social engineering etc."

48. Wikipedia: Herbert Ley, Jr. Quote from San Francisco Chronicle article of January 2, 1970. Retrieved March 18, 2008, http://en.wikipedia.org/wiki/Herbert_Ley,_Jr.

49. Emily Friedman. "Happy Tails, Jake Leg, and the Food and Drug Administration."

Appendix II

HHN Magazine online, August 7, 2007; retrieved March 2008 http://www.
hhnmag.com/hhnmag_app/jsp/articledisplay.jsp?dcrpath=HHNMAG/Article/
data/08AUG2007/070807HHN_Online_Friedman&domain=HHNMAG

Citations, Chapter 2—

1. Lauren Streib. "World's Fattest Countries." Forbes, Health, 02.08.07, http://www.forbes.
    com/2007/02/07/worlds-fattest-countries-forbeslife-cx_ls_0208worldfat.html

2. David Rumbach. "Growing numbers." South Bend Tribune, May 28, 2006, http://www.
    southbendtribune.com/apps/pbcs.dll/article?AID=/20060528/News01/605280407/-1/
    NEWS01/CAT=News01

3. Obesity Action Coalition. "Understanding Morbid Obesity." OAC Web site, retrieved
    02/08/08, http://www.obesityaction.org/educationaltools/brochures/uoseries/umo.php

4. Amanda Gardner. "Eating Out Doesn't Guarantee Weight Gain But fast food is no friend
    of the waistline, new study finds." U.S.News & World Report, Health, Posted 1/21/08,
    http://health.usnews.com/usnews/health/healthday/080121/eating-out-doesnt-guarantee-
    weight-gain.htm

5. Peter Singer, Jim Mason. "The Way We Eat, why our food choices matter." Rodale Books;
    May 2, 2006, p. 280. They quoted from: Judy Putnam, "US Food Supply Providing More
    Food and Calories, " FoodReview, vol. 22, no.3 (Sept 1999), Table 1, p. 6; http://www.ers.
    usda.gov/publication/foodreview/spt1999/frsept99a.pdf

6. Karl Niedershuh. "The World's Heaviest People." Dimensions Magazine, retrieved
    03/08/08, http://www.dimensionsmagazine.com/dimtext/kjn/people/heaviest.htm

7. Lori Weaver. "Distillers grains can be good choice for poultry." Feed Industry Network.
    com, Aug 18, 2008 This article appeared in Feed Management, November 2007, http://
    www.feedindustrynetwork.com/0711FMPoultry.aspx

8. Karl Loren. "Most Americans Take Medication Weekly; Many Take Multiple Products."
    Vibrant Life, from JAMA. (Journal of the American Medical Association) 2002;287:337-
    344, January 16 issue, http://www.chelationtherapyonline.com/articles/p67.htm

9. Jennifer Harper. "Overweight but unconcerned; chubby, tubby, portly, stout: Americans
    may be more at home with a little extra padding, or so, these days." Insight on the
    News, August 19, 2002, http://findarticles.com/p/articles/mi_m1571/is_30_18/
    ai_90753055/?tag=content;col1

10. EmilyH. "Fat War Misses a Couple of Marks." Big Fat Blog, January 12th, 2007, http://
    www.bigfatblog.com/node/1328

11. Margaret Adamek, PhD. "Kicking the Habit." Excerpted from a workshop presentation
    at the 2005 Bioneers Conference; retrieved 2008, http://www.bioneers.org/node/2263

12. The Food Allergy & Anaphylaxis Network. "Increase in students with food allergies." 24
    August 2005, retrieved from The Medical News, Child Health News, 2008, http://www.
    news-medical.net/news/2005/08/24/12678.aspx

13. Jane E. Brody. "Forget the Second Helpings. It's the First Ones That Count." The New
    York Times, Personal Health, July 11, 2006, http://www.nytimes.com/2006/07/11/health/
    nutrition/11brody.html

14. "Obesity, psychiatric disorders go hand in hand: new study." China View, Health, 2006-
    07-05, http://news.xinhuanet.com/english/2006-07/05/content_4796272.htm

15. Brad Lemley. "What Does Science Say You Should Eat?" Discover, Health & Medicine/ Obesity, 02.05.2004, http://discovermagazine.com/2004/feb/science-diet/

16. "Diabetes Mellitus", Encyclopedia Americana, Library Edition, vol. 9, 1966, pp. 54-56, retrieved from: Tom Smith, for Nexus Magazine, Volume 11, Number 4 (June-July 2004) http://www.whale.to/a/smith.html

17. Op. cit., Discover, Health & Medicine/ Obesity.

18. "Pregnancy and Pica: Non-Food Cravings." American Pregnancy Association. Last Updated: 03/2007, retrieved 2008, http://www.americanpregnancy.org/pregnancyhealth/unusualcravingspica.html

19. Op. cit., "The Way We Eat, why our food choices matter." p.59

20. Donald L. Barlett And James B. Steele, "Monsanto's Harvest of Fear." Vanity Fair, May 2008, p. 2 http://www.vanityfair.com/politics/features/2008/05/monsanto200805?currentPage=2

21. Rebecca Tushnet. "Playing chicken: "raised without antibiotics" draws lawsuit." Rebecca Tushnet's 43(B)log/ False advertising and more, April 18, 2008, http://tushnet.blogspot.com/2008/04/playing-chicken-raised-without.html

22. Film: "Life Running Out of Control." Directed by Bertram Verhaag, produced by Michel Morales and Bertram Verhaag for DENKmal-Films and Haifisch Films 2004, aired 2008 on LinkTV; see http://www.linktv.org/

Citations, Chapter 3—

1. Suzanne Hamlin. "Can't Cook? I Mean, Really Can't Cook?" The New York Times, Home & Garden, August 7, 1996. http://www.nytimes.com/1996/08/07/garden/can-t-cook-i-mean-really-can-t-cook.html

2. Robert Ebbin. "Americans' Dining-Out Habits." National Restaurant Association, Restaurants USA online, November 2000. http://www.restaurant.org/rusa/magArticle.cfm?ArticleID=138

3. Martin Stack. "A Concise History of America's Brewing Industry". EH.Net Encyclopedia, edited by Robert Whaples. July 4, 2003. http://eh.net/encyclopedia/article/stack.brewing.industry.history.us

4. Chowhound message board, Spirits/ Whiskey, Bourbon, Tequila, Rum, and Other Distilled Potables, Oct 23, 2007, http://chowhound.chow.com/topics/453167

5. Wikipedia. Jamaican ginger, retrieved April 18, 2008, http://en.wikipedia.org/wiki/Jamaican_ginger

6. Janet L. Allured. "Women's Healing Art: Domestic Medicine in the Turn-of-the-Century Ozarks." Spring 1992 issue of Gateway Heritage , vol. 12, no. 4, Missouri Historical Society, Bernard Becker Medical Library, Washington University School of Medicine, St. Louis, Missouri. http://beckerexhibits.wustl.edu/mowihsp/articles/Ozarks.htm

7. Isadora Stehlin. "Homeopathy: Real Medicine or Empty Promises?" FDA Consumer magazine (December 1996), US Food and Drug Administration. http://www.fda.gov/fdac/features/096_home.html

8. Dana Ullman, M.P.H. "A Condensed History Of Homeopathy." Excerpted from Discovering Homeopathy: Medicine for the 21st Century, published by Berkeley: North Atlantic, 1995. http://www.healthy.net/scr/Article.asp?Id=860

9. Wellness Directory of Minnesota. "The History of Medicine 1800 – 1850." 2003, retrieved 4/19/08; http://www.mnwelldir.org/docs/history/history03.htm

10. Lawrence D. Wilson, M.D. "Healing the Health-Care System." The Future of Freedom Foundation, Freedom Daily, December 2001. http://www.fff.org/freedom/1201e.asp

11. Barbara Ehrenreich and Deirdre English. "Witches, Midwives, and Nurses: A History of Women Healers." From the archives of The Memory Hole, Originally published by The Feminist Press at CUNY. 11 Nov 2004. http://tmh.floonet.net/articles/witches.html

12. Dexter Tiranti. "A Pill for Every Ill." The New Internationalist, New Internationalist issue 165 - November 1986. http://www.newint.org/issue165/keynote.htm

13. Thomas Hine. Populuxe. (New York; Alfred A. Knopf, 1987), p. 27

Citations, Chapter 4—

1. Amy Levek ,"Uranium Cuts a Tragic Path Through the Navajo Nation." Turtle Talk, Blog at WordPress.com, retrieved August 2008 http://turtletalk.wordpress. com/2008/01/03/news-article-on-uranium-mining-impact-at-navajo/

2. Seven Deadly Sins website: http://www.deadlysins.com/sins/, retrieved August 2008.

3. Patricia Gothard, Laguna Woods, CA, 2008; in response to BBC editorial by Peter Baker. "Feeling the heat of food security." *BBC News*, 11 August 2008, retrieved August 2008. http://news.bbc.co.uk/2/hi/science/nature/7553958.stm

Citations, Chapter 5—

1. Fran Henry. "Factory Farms Cause Big "Stink." Cleveland Plain Dealer, August 01, 2004; retrieved October 2008 from Organic Consumers Association, http://www. organicconsumers.org/corp/stink081104.cfm

2. Aly Adair. "Bottled Beverages - Where Will We Waste Them?" Associated Content, Business & Finance, May 18, 2007, retrieved November 2008. http://www. associatedcontent.com/article/245990/bottled_beverages_where_will_we_waste. html?cat=3

3. ScienceDaily. "Drink Brewed Tea To Avoid Tooth Erosion, Study Suggests." Science News, Nov. 28, 2008, retrieved November 2008. http://www.sciencedaily.com/ releases/2008/11/081125132514.htm

4. Environmental Defense Fund. "Fighting Global Warming with Food." Posted: 24-Jul-2007; Updated: 27-Aug-2007. Retrieved September 2008. http://www.edf.org/article. cfm?contentid=6604

5. All organic ingredients, and what I paid for them in 2008:
    Whole wheat pasta 14oz, 4 servings (they claim 7) @ 2.99= .75 per serving
    Dried chickpeas 16oz, 8 servings (they say 10) @ 3.42= .42 per serving
    Fresh snow peas 1 lb, 13.3 servings (from a food site) @ 7.70/lb.= .58 per serving
    Garlic bulbs, ½ lb = 4 bulbs, roughly= 2.50/ bulb =.62 per serving
    Olive oil 25oz, 25 servings (my est.) @ 10 bottle= .40 per serving
    Total= $2.77 per person.

6. MIStupid.com. "Stupid Facts - Pasta Names" Retrieved October 2008. http://mistupid. com/facts/page047.htm

7. Tom Philpott. "Meet the Lunch Lady: Maverick Chef Ann Cooper Aims to Spark a Nationwide School-Lunch Revolution." Grist Magazine, Jan 18, 2007; retrieved from the Organic Consumers Association, October 2008. http://www.organicconsumers.org/articles/article_3865.cfm

8. Ann Cooper. "Katie Wilson's Testimony." Chef Ann Cooper Blog, July 9, 2008, retrieved July 21, 2008. http://www.chefann.com/blog/archives/1018

9. The Physicians Committee for Responsible Medicine (PCRM). "School Lunches Labeled "Weapons of Mass Destruction" in Provocative New Ad." PCRM News and Media Center, News Release, October 7, 2002. Retrieved July 21, 2008. http://www.pcrm.org/news/health021007.html

10. Ann Hulbert. "I Say the Hell With It!" Slate, Sandbox: Keeping an Eye on Kids and Parents, posted Feb. 11, 2003, retrieved July 2008. http://www.slate.com/id/2078416/

11. Tom Cullison. "School Food Environments: Then and Now." School Nutrition Association, SNA News, posted July 9, 2008, retrieved July 2008. http://www.schoolnutrition.org/Blog.aspx?id=9876&blogid=622

12. Amelia Buragas. "Women increasingly are choosing artisan and industrial cheesemaking as career path." The Cooperative Extension System, extension.org. Posted August 29, 2007, retrieved July 2008. http://www.extension.org/pages/Women_increasingly_are_choosing_artisan_and_industrial_cheesemaking_as_career_path

13. Clarke Historical Library, Central Michigan University, "Michigan Cookbooks: 150 Years of Mostly Good Meals"; taken from Lovegren, Fashionable Food, 170. Retrieved July 2008. http://clarke.cmich.edu/cookbookscatalog/catalog3.htm

14. Beaver Club of Lafayette, Incorporated. Cajun Men Cook: Recipes, Stories and Food Experiences from Louisiana Cajun Country, December 1994; Text taken from website pages, July 2008. http://www.cajunmencook.com/cook/

15. Website: Advantour- Silk Road/ Central Asia/ Uzbekistan: Culture. Published 2001-2008, retrieved July 2008. http://www.advantour.com/uzbekistan/culture.htm

16. Elaine Louie. "Tamales Are Hot, As in Popular." The New York Times, Dining & Wine, May 22, 2002. Retrieved July 2008. http://www.nytimes.com/2002/05/22/dining/tamales-are-hot-as-in-popular.html

17. Lisa Fain, The Homesick Texan. "Let's Make Tamales: Part 1." Homesick Texan blog, posted November 30, 2006, retrieved July 2008. http://homesicktexan.blogspot.com/search/label/lard

18. Hawaii: Village Houses, Polynesian Cultural Center website, Cooking implements, retrieved July 2008, http://www.polynesia.com/hawaii/village-houses.html

19. Barbara Fisher. "Is Cooking For Your Family "Retrograde June Cleaver Nonsense?" Tigers & Strawberries, a food blog, posted July 16, 2007, retrieved July 2008. http://www.tigersandstrawberries.com/2007/07/16/is-cooking-for-your-family-retrograde-june-cleaver-nonsense/

20. Sue Carswell. "A Conversation with Dara Torres." Women's Health, Life section, posted October 7, 2008, retrieved October 2008. http://www.womenshealthmag.com/life/meet-dara-torres

Appendix II

Citations, Chapter 6—

1. Meera. "Kshamavaani Day or kshama Divas of Jain People." Festivals in India website, posted March 13th, 2006, retrieved August 2008. http://www.festivalsindia.com/kshamavaani-day-or-kshama-divas-of-jain-people/

   Also, Wikipedia: Kshamavaani. Retrieved August 2008. http://en.wikipedia.org/wiki/Kshamavaani

2. Center for Food Safety website. "Sewage Sludge." Retrieved April 2008. http://www.centerforfoodsafety.org/sewage_slu.cfm

3. Jonathan Bloom. "The food not eaten." Culinate (website), November 19, 2007, retrieved April 2008. http://www.culinate.com/articles/features/wasted_food

4. Environment News Service. "Half the American Harvest Goes to Waste." ENS-News, November 23, 2004, retrieved May 2008. http://www.ens-newswire.com/ens/nov2004/2004-11-23-04.asp

5. Andrew Martin. "One Country's Table Scraps, Another Country's Meal." *The New York Times*, The World, Week in Review, May 18, 2008. http://www.nytimes.com/2008/05/18/weekinreview/18martin.html?_r=1

6. Tom Mosakowski. "Estrogen Mimicry of Bisphenol-A Threatens Human and Animal Health." Natural News.com, March 17, 2008, retrieved August 2008. http://www.naturalnews.com/022848.html

7. National Heart, Lung and Blood Institute website. "Portion Distortion Interactive Quiz." National Institutes of Health, Department of Health and Human Services; retrieved May 2008. http://hp2010.nhlbihin.net/portion/index.htm

8. FamilyEducation.com, "Calorie Guidelines for Women." Family Education Network. Retrieved June 2008. http://life.familyeducation.com/nutrition-and-diet/weight/35881.html

9. WebMD, LLC. in collaboration with the Cleveland Clinic. "Portion Control and Weight Loss." WebMD.com, Healthy Eating & Diet. Retrieved August 2008. http://www.webmd.com/diet/control-portion-size

10. Beverly Hassell. "Sauerkraut contains anticancer compound." American Chemical Society, 17-Oct-2002, retrieved from Eurekalert.org, August 2008. http://www.eurekalert.org/pub_releases/2002-10/acs-sca101702.php

11. Wikipedia: Fermentation (Food). Retrieved August 2008. http://en.wikipedia.org/wiki/Fermentation_(food)

12. James T. Ehler. "American Customs Quotes." Food Reference.com, Quotes section, Food Quotes. Retrieved September 2008. http://www.foodreference.com/html/q-american-customs.html

13. CNBC Original Special, reported by Melissa Lee. "Made in China: The People's Republic of Profit." Aired on CNBC August 3, 2008. http://www.cnbc.com/id/25921229/

14. Robert Krulwich. "Sweet, Sour, Salty, Bitter ... and Umami." National Public Radio, *Morning Edition,* November 5, 2007, NPR.com. Retrieved September 2008. http://www.npr.org/templates/story/story.php?storyId=15819485

Citations, Chapter 7—

1. Jonah Lehrer. "How the city hurts your brain …And what you can do about it." *Boston Globe*, Ideas section, January 2, 2009; retrieved January 2009 http://www.boston. com/bostonglobe/ideas/articles/2009/01/04/how_the_city_hurts_your_brain/

2. Susan Brink. "Sing Out, Sister." *Los Angeles Times*, Health section, April 23, 2007, retrieved January 2009. http://articles.latimes.com/2007/apr/23/health/he-sing23

3. SixWise.com. "How Singing Improves Your Health." Newsletter June 7, 2006; retrieved January 2009 http://www.sixwise.com/newsletters/06/06/07/how_singing_improves_your_health_even_if_other_people_shouldnt_hear_you_singing.htm

    "Several studies have found that singing also enhances immunity and well-being. One, conducted at the University of Frankfurt in Germany, found that choral members had higher levels of immunoglobulin A and cortisol -- markers of enhanced immunity -- after they sang Mozart's "Requiem" than before. Just listening to the music did not have this effect."

4. John Sparks. "The Singing-Health Connection A growing body of research demonstrates enhanced health and emotional benefits." *The Voice*, Chorus America, Winter 2004-05; retrieved January 2009 http://chorusamerica.org/vox_article_singinghealth.cfm

5. Bio-Medicine.org. "Singing Leads to Better Health." Medicine, News, 11/30/2005; retrieved January 2009 http://www.bio-medicine.org/medicine-news/Singing-Leads-To-Better-Health-5971-1/

www.worshipyourfood.com

www.ingramcontent.com/pod-product-compliance
Lightning Source LLC
Chambersburg PA
CBHW031508270326
41930CB00006B/304